MILITARY AND VETERAN ISSUES

RECOVERING SERVICEMEMBERS AND VETERANS

ASSESSMENTS OF CARE AND BENEFITS MANAGEMENT

Military and Veteran Issues

Additional books in this series can be found on Nova's website under the Series tab.

Additional E-books in this series can be found on Nova's website under the E-book tab.

Health Care Issues, Costs and Access

Additional books in this series can be found on Nova's website under the Series tab.

Additional E-books in this series can be found on Nova's website under the E-book tab.

MILITARY AND VETERAN ISSUES

RECOVERING SERVICEMEMBERS AND VETERANS

ASSESSMENTS OF CARE AND BENEFITS MANAGEMENT

IRA WACHTEL
AND
GINA NUTTING
EDITORS

nova publishers
New York

For permission to use material from this book please contact us:
Telephone 631-231-7269; Fax 631-231-8175
Web Site: http://www.novapublishers.com

Library of Congress Cataloging-in-Publication Data

ISBN: 978-1-62417-775-0

Published by Nova Science Publishers, Inc. † New York

CONTENTS

PREFACE

Deficiencies exposed at Walter Reed Army Medical Center in 2007 served as a catalyst compelling the Departments of Defense (DoD) and Veterans Affairs (VA) to address a host of problems for wounded, ill, and injured servicemembers and veterans as they navigate through the recovery care continuum. This continuum extends from acute medical treatment and stabilization, through rehabilitation to reintegration, either back to active duty or to the civilian community as a veteran. In spite of 5 years of departmental efforts, recovering servicemembers and veterans are still facing problems with this process and may not be getting the services they need. This book provides an overview and assessment of the care and benefit management system for recovering servicemembers and veterans.

Chapter 1 – The National Defense Authorization Act for Fiscal Year 2008 required DOD and VA to jointly develop and implement policy on the care, management, and transition of recovering servicemembers. It also required GAO to report on DOD's and VA's progress in addressing these requirements. This report specifically examines (1) the extent to which DOD and VA have resolved persistent problems facing recovering servicemembers and veterans as they navigate the recovery care continuum, and (2) the reasons DOD and VA leadership have not been able to fully resolve any remaining problems. To address these objectives, GAO visited 11 DOD and VA medical facilities selected for population size and range of available resources and met with servicemembers and veterans to identify problems they continue to face. GAO also reviewed documents related to specific DOD and VA programs that assist recovering servicemembers and veterans and interviewed the leadership and staff of these programs to determine why problems have not been fully resolved.

Chapter 2 - Since 2007, DOD and VA have jointly operated IDES—which is intended to expedite benefits for injured servicemembers. IDES replaced the departments' separate processes for evaluating servicemembers for fitness and disability. Initially a pilot at 3 military treatment facilities, IDES is now in place at military treatment facilities worldwide. In previous reports, GAO identified a number of challenges as IDES expanded to more facilities, including staffing shortages and difficultly meeting timeliness goals.

In light of IDES' expansion, GAO was asked to examine: (1) the extent to which DOD and VA are meeting IDES timeliness and servicemember satisfaction performance goals, and (2) steps the agencies are taking to improve IDES performance. GAO analyzed IDES timeliness and customer satisfaction data, visited six IDES sites with varying performance, and interviewed DOD and VA officials.

In: Recovering Servicemembers and Veterans ISBN: 978-1-62417-775-0
Editors: Ira Wachtel and Gina Nutting

Chapter 1

RECOVERING SERVICEMEMBERS AND VETERANS: SUSTAINED LEADERSHIP ATTENTION AND SYSTEMATIC OVERSIGHT NEEDED TO RESOLVE PERSISTENT PROBLEMS AFFECTING CARE AND BENEFITS*

United States Government Accountability Office

ABBREVIATIONS

DOD	Department of Defense
Dole-Shalala Commission	President's Commission on Care for America's Returning Wounded Warriors
FRCP	Federal Recovery Coordination Program
IDES	Integrated disability evaluation system
LOA	Line of Action
MTF	military treatment facility
NDAA 2008	National Defense Authorization Act for Fiscal Year 2008

* This is an edited, reformatted and augmented version of The United States Government Accountability Office publication, Report to Congressional Committees, GAO-13-5, dated November 2012.

OEF	Operation Enduring Freedom
OIF	Operation Iraqi Freedom
OND	Operation New Dawn
PTSD	posttraumatic stress disorder
RCP	Recovery Coordination Program
Recovering Warrior Task Force	Department of Defense Task Force on the Care, Management, and Transition of Recovering Wounded, Ill, and Injured Members of the Armed Forces
Senior Oversight Committee	Wounded, Ill, and Injured Senior Oversight Committee
TBI	traumatic brain injury
VA	Department of Veterans Affairs
VAMC	Department of Veterans Affairs Medical Center
WWCTP	Office of Wounded Warrior Care and Transition Policy

WHY GAO DID THIS STUDY

The National Defense Authorization Act for Fiscal Year 2008 required DOD and VA to jointly develop and implement policy on the care, management, and transition of recovering servicemembers. It also required GAO to report on DOD's and VA's progress in addressing these requirements. This report specifically examines (1) the extent to which DOD and VA have resolved persistent problems facing recovering servicemembers and veterans as they navigate the recovery care continuum, and (2) the reasons DOD and VA leadership have not been able to fully resolve any remaining problems. To address these objectives, GAO visited 11 DOD and VA medical facilities selected for population size and range of available resources and met with servicemembers and veterans to identify problems they continue to face.

GAO also reviewed documents related to specific DOD and VA programs that assist recovering servicemembers and veterans and interviewed the leadership and staff of these programs to determine why problems have not been fully resolved.

WHAT GAO RECOMMENDS

GAO recommends that DOD provide central oversight of the military services' wounded warrior programs and that DOD and VA sustain high-level leadership attention and collaboration to fully resolve identified problems. DOD partially concurred with the recommendation for central oversight of the wounded warrior programs, citing issues with common eligibility criteria and systematic monitoring. DOD and VA both concurred with the recommendation for sustained leadership attention.

WHAT GAO FOUND

Deficiencies exposed at Walter Reed Army Medical Center in 2007 served as a catalyst compelling the Departments of Defense (DOD) and Veterans Affairs (VA) to address a host of problems for wounded, ill, and injured servicemembers and veterans as they navigate through the recovery care continuum. This continuum extends from acute medical treatment and stabilization, through rehabilitation to reintegration, either back to active duty or to the civilian community as a veteran. In spite of 5 years of departmental efforts, recovering servicemembers and veterans are still facing problems with this process and may not be getting the services they need. Key departmental efforts included the creation or modification of various care coordination and case management programs, including the military services' wounded warrior programs. However, these programs are not always accessible to those who need them due to the inconsistent methods, such as referrals, used to identify potentially eligible servicemembers, as well as inconsistent eligibility criteria across the military services' wounded warrior programs. The departments also jointly established an integrated disability evaluation system to expedite the delivery of benefits to servicemembers. However, processing times for disability determinations under the new system have increased since 2007, resulting in lengthy wait times that limit servicemembers' ability to plan for their future. Finally, despite years of incremental efforts, DOD and VA have yet to develop sufficient capabilities for electronically sharing complete health records, which potentially delays servicemembers' receipt of coordinated care and benefits as they transition from DOD's to VA's health care system.

Collectively, a lack of leadership, oversight, resources, and collaboration has contributed to the departments' inability to fully resolve problems facing recovering servicemembers and veterans. Initially, departmental leadership exhibited focus and commitment—through the Senior Oversight Committee—to addressing problems related to case management and care coordination, disability evaluation systems, and data sharing between DOD and VA. However, the committee's oversight waned over time, and in January 2012, it was merged with the VA/DOD Joint Executive Council. Whether this council—which has primarily focused on long-term strategic planning—can effectively address the shorter-term policy focused issues once managed by the Senior Oversight Committee remains to be seen. Furthermore, DOD does not provide central oversight of the military services' wounded warrior programs, preventing it from determining how well these programs are working across the department. However, despite these shortcomings, the departments continue to take steps to resolve identified problems, such as increasing the number of staff involved with the electronic sharing of health records and the integrated disability evaluation process. Additionally, while the departments' previous attempts to collaborate on how to resolve case management and care coordination problems have largely been unsuccessful, a joint task force established in May 2012 is focused on resolving long-standing areas of disagreement between VA, DOD, and the military services. However, without more robust oversight and military service compliance, consistent implementation of policies that result in more effective case management and care coordination programs may be unattainable.

November 16, 2012

Congressional Committees

A series of media reports in early 2007 disclosed troublesome deficiencies in the provision of outpatient services at Walter Reed Army Medical Center in Washington, D.C.[1] These reports prompted broader questions about whether the Departments of Defense (DOD) and Veterans Affairs (VA) were fully prepared to meet the needs of the growing number of servicemembers and veterans returning from recent conflicts. Several review groups were subsequently tasked with investigating the reported problems and identifying recommendations.[2] These groups identified common areas of concern including: inadequate case management to ensure continuity of care,[3] confusing disability evaluation systems, and insufficient sharing of servicemembers' health records and other data between DOD and VA—all long-standing problems that we have reported on extensively.[4]

To elevate the response to concerns raised by these review groups, DOD and VA established the Wounded, Ill, and Injured Senior Oversight Committee (Senior Oversight Committee) in May 2007. The committee was intended to operate on a short-term basis to review and implement the recommendations made by the various review groups and improve seamlessness in the provision of care for recovering servicemembers and veterans.[5] It was cochaired by the Deputy Secretaries of Defense and Veterans Affairs and included the military service Secretaries and other high-ranking officials within the departments. Congress subsequently passed the National Defense Authorization Act for Fiscal Year 2008 (NDAA 2008) requiring the Secretary of Defense and the Secretary of Veterans Affairs to jointly develop and implement policy, to the extent feasible, to improve the care, management, and transition of recovering servicemembers.[6] Because of its related ongoing work, the Senior Oversight Committee also assumed responsibility for addressing these requirements.

Despite actions taken by DOD and VA to address the problems identified at Walter Reed in 2007, concerns remain that recovering servicemembers and veterans continue to face many of the same problems as they did in 2007 navigating the recovery care continuum, from acute medical treatment and stabilization, through rehabilitation, to reintegration—either back to active duty or to the civilian community as a veteran. In 2009, Congress required DOD to establish a task force to assess the effectiveness of DOD programs and policies developed to assist recovering servicemembers and to make recommendations for continuous improvements of such policies and programs.[7] The DOD Task Force on the Care, Management, and Transition of Recovering Wounded, Ill, and Injured Members of the Armed Forces—referred to as the Recovering Warrior Task Force—issued its first report in September 2011;[8] it contained 21 recommendations on a variety of issues affecting recovering servicemembers.[9] Additionally, congressional committees held multiple hearings in 2010 and 2011 that highlighted ongoing difficulties facing these servicemembers and veterans, including issues with duplication and poor coordination among case management and care coordination programs,[10] delays in completing the disability evaluation process, and the lack of full interoperability between DOD's and VA's computer systems.[11]

The NDAA 2008 required that we report on DOD's and VA's progress in developing and implementing joint policy on issues related to the care, management, and transition of recovering servicemembers.[12] As discussed with the committees of jurisdiction, we have reviewed and reported on the departments' progress with respect to various topic areas. This review, which is focused on the continuity of care for recovering servicemembers and veterans, is the latest in our body of work.[13] In this review, we are reporting on

1) the extent to which DOD and VA have resolved persistent problems facing recovering servicemembers and veterans as they navigate the recovery care continuum and
2) the reasons DOD and VA leadership have not been able to fully resolve any remaining problems.

To respond to these objectives, we interviewed the directors of the following case management and care coordination programs,[14] including

- the Army Warrior Care and Transition Command's Warrior Transition Units and the Army Wounded Warrior Program,
- the Navy Safe Harbor Program,
- the Air Force Recovery Care Program and the Air Force Wounded Warrior Program,
- the Marine Corps Wounded Warrior Regiment,
- the United States Special Operations Command's Care Coalition,
- the Federal Recovery Coordination Program, and
- VA's Operation Enduring Freedom/Operation Iraqi Freedom/ Operation New Dawn (OEF/OIF/OND) Care Management Program.

We collected data for each of these programs, such as the number of enrollees over time. (See app. I for data on enrollment and population characteristics for these programs.) We also reviewed documents describing the scope, mission, and leadership of these selected programs.

In addition, we took the following steps to determine the extent to which DOD and VA have resolved persistent problems affecting recovering servicemembers and veterans along the recovery care continuum:

- We visited a judgmental sample of 11 DOD military treatment facilities (MTF) and VA Medical Centers (VAMC) to identify variations in how care coordination and case management programs are being operated at the local level. We focused on Army and Marine Corps MTFs because, collectively, the wounded warrior programs for these military services serve more than 70 percent of the wounded, ill, and injured servicemember and veteran population. We selected facilities that provide or have access to significant medical and rehabilitation resources as well as facilities that have fewer medical or rehabilitation resources. The sites we visited included MTFs at Fort Bragg (N.C.), Fort Knox (Ky.), Fort Carson (Colo.), Fort Belvoir (Va.), Fort Meade (Md.), Walter Reed National Military Medical Center (Md.), Camp Lejeune (N.C.), and Quantico (Va.), and VAMCs in Richmond, Virginia; Denver, Colorado; and the District of Columbia. At these facilities, we met with local leadership officials and the officials responsible for managing the facilities' case management and care coordination programs, and we obtained information on how these programs were working as well as the types of problems that recovering servicemembers and veterans continue to face. While at these facilities, we met with recovering servicemembers and veterans to obtain information about their experiences.

- We interviewed officials from military and veteran advocacy groups to obtain their members' perspective on any problems that persist in navigating the recovery care continuum.
- We interviewed the director of the VA Liaison for Healthcare Program to understand VA's role in assisting recovering servicemembers' transition from DOD's to VA's health care system.
- We met with members of the Recovering Warrior Task Force, reviewed relevant task force documentation, and attended its public meetings to obtain information about problems they identified that affect recovering servicemembers and veterans.
- We reviewed published and ongoing studies and GAO reports[15] describing problems that recovering servicemembers and veterans face, including issues related to the disability evaluation system and the electronic sharing of health records between DOD and VA.

To identify the reasons why DOD and VA leadership have not fully resolved any remaining problems facing recovering servicemembers and veterans, we reviewed relevant documentation to identify the roles of DOD and VA offices that coordinate or oversee case management or care coordination programs, their placement within their respective departments, and whether and how these offices monitor the performance of the programs we reviewed. We also obtained information about organizational and program changes, including officials' views about the potential impact of these changes.

We also interviewed key DOD and VA leadership officials, such as the Deputy Assistant Secretary of Defense for Wounded Warrior Care and Transition Policy, VA's Chief of Staff, and former and current officials from the departments' coordinating and oversight offices, including the Senior Oversight Committee, DOD's Office of Wounded Warrior Care and Transition Policy, the Interagency Program Office, and the VA/DOD Collaboration Service, which is an office within VA.

To obtain information about recent efforts DOD and VA have initiated to address problems facing servicemembers and veterans, we interviewed DOD and VA officials participating in these activities, including officials involved in the DOD and VA Warrior Care and Coordination Taskforce. We also reviewed the documentation available regarding the departments' recent efforts; however, we predominately relied on testimonial evidence provided by these officials.

The NDAA 2008 also requires us to certify whether we had timely access to sufficient information to make informed judgments on the matters covered by our report.

We were provided sufficient information in a timely manner to assess the extent to which DOD and VA have resolved persistent problems facing recovering servicemembers and veterans as they navigate the recovery care continuum and the reasons DOD and VA leadership have not been able to fully resolve any remaining problems.

We conducted this performance audit from July 2011 through September 2012 in accordance with generally accepted government auditing standards. Those standards require that we plan and perform the audit to obtain sufficient, appropriate evidence to provide a reasonable basis for our findings and conclusions based on our audit objectives. We believe that the evidence obtained provides a reasonable basis for our findings and conclusions based on our audit objectives.

BACKGROUND

Review groups identified significant problems after the media reports concerning Walter Reed.

Initial efforts to respond to these problems were primarily coordinated through the Senior Oversight Committee, and DOD and VA undertook additional efforts to respond to these problems.

Review Groups Identified Problems across the Recovery Care Continuum

Following the revelations at Walter Reed, several review groups noted significant problems that may arise during servicemembers' recovery from wounds, illnesses, and injuries.[16] Some of these problems involve the provision of appropriate medical care, while others involve the acquisition of needed DOD and VA benefits. In 2007, one of the review groups, the President's Commission on Care for America's Returning Wounded Warriors—commonly referred to as the Dole-Shalala Commission—noted that recovering servicemembers depend on the effective and efficient provision of medical services and benefits across the recovery care continuum,[17] which is separated into three phases:

- *recovery*, when wounded, ill, and injured servicemembers are stabilized and receive acute inpatient medical treatment at an MTF, VAMC, or private medical facility;
- *rehabilitation*, when recovering servicemembers with complex trauma, such as missing limbs, receive medical and rehabilitative care; and
- *reintegration*, when servicemembers either return to active duty or to the civilian community as veterans.

A recovering servicemember or veteran may not experience the recovery care continuum as a linear process, and may move back and forth across the continuum over time, depending on his or her medical needs. For example, a servicemember who has transitioned to the rehabilitation phase may go back to the recovery phase if there is a need to return to an MTF to obtain acute medical care, such as a surgical procedure.

Initial Efforts to Address Problems Were Coordinated by the Senior Oversight Committee

DOD and VA took a number of steps to address the problems identified by the review groups that investigated the issues raised by the Walter Reed media reports. As an initial step, the departments established the Senior Oversight Committee to coordinate and oversee DOD's and VA's efforts to jointly resolve these problems. Through this committee, DOD and VA created programs and initiatives to assist recovering servicemembers and veterans as they navigate the recovery care continuum. Key efforts included the establishment of the integrated disability evaluation system (IDES), the Federal Recovery Coordination Program (FRCP), the Recovery Coordination Program (RCP), and the Interagency Program Office. (See fig. 1.)

Senior Oversight Committee. The Senior Oversight Committee was responsible for ensuring that the recommendations—which totaled more than 600 from the various review groups—were properly reviewed, coordinated, implemented, and resourced.

Supporting the Senior Oversight Committee was an Overarching Integrated Product Team, the membership of which included the Assistant Secretaries of Defense, the military departments' Assistant Secretaries for Manpower and Reserve Affairs, and various senior officials from DOD and VA. This team coordinated, integrated, and synchronized the work of the eight "Lines of Action" (LOA) that focused on specific issues, including case management, disability evaluation systems, and data sharing between DOD and VA. (See fig. 2.)

Each LOA included representation from DOD, including each military service, and VA. They performed the bulk of the work to address the issues and recommendations of the various review groups, including establishing plans, setting and tracking milestones, and identifying and enacting early and short-term solutions. More specifically, the LOAs were as follows:

- *LOA 1*—Disability Evaluation: Responsible for addressing efforts to reform the DOD and VA disability evaluation systems.
- *LOA 2*—Traumatic Brain Injury (TBI)/Post Traumatic Stress Disorder (PTSD): Responsible for addressing issues related to TBI/PTSD.
- *LOA 3*—Case Management: Responsible for addressing issues related to the care, management, and transition of recovering servicemembers from recovery to rehabilitation and reintegration.
- *LOA 4*—DOD/VA Data Sharing: Responsible for addressing issues regarding the electronic exchange of DOD and VA health records.
- *LOA 5*—Facilities: Responsible for addressing issues relating to military and VA medical facilities.
- *LOA 6*—"Clean Sheet" Review: Developed recommendations to improve care and benefits without the constraints of existing laws, regulations, organizational roles, personnel constraints, or budgets.

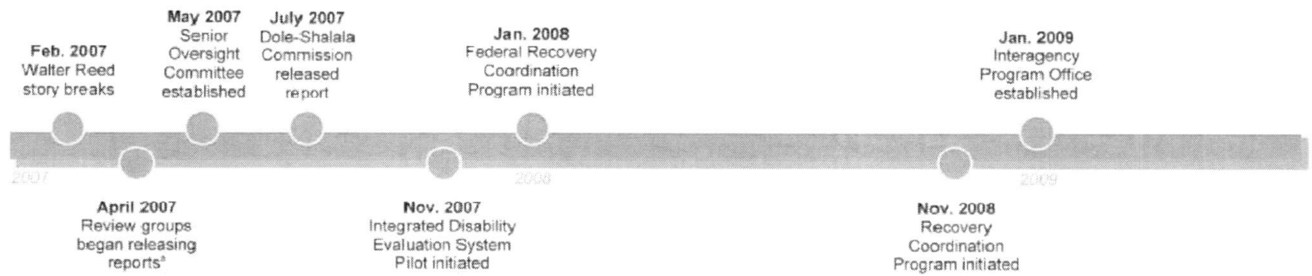

Source: Department of Defense.

[a] Several review groups, including the Dole-Shalala Commission, were tasked with investigating the problems reported at Walter Reed Army Medical Center in Washington, D.C., and identifying recommendations. The other review groups included the Independent Review Group, Rebuilding the Trust: Report on Rehabilitative Care and Administrative Processes at Walter Reed Army Medical Center and National Naval Medical Center (Arlington, Va.: April 2007); Task Force on Returning Global War on Terror Heroes, Report to the President (April 2007); Veterans' Disability Benefits Commission, Honoring the Call to Duty: Veterans' Disability Benefits in the 21st Century (October 2007); and Department of Defense Office of the Inspector General, Department of Veterans Affairs Office of the Inspector General, DOD/VA Care Transition Process for Service Members Injured in OIF/OEF (June 2008).

Figure 1. Timeline of Key Events in the 2-Year Period Following the Walter Reed Army Medical Center Media Reports.

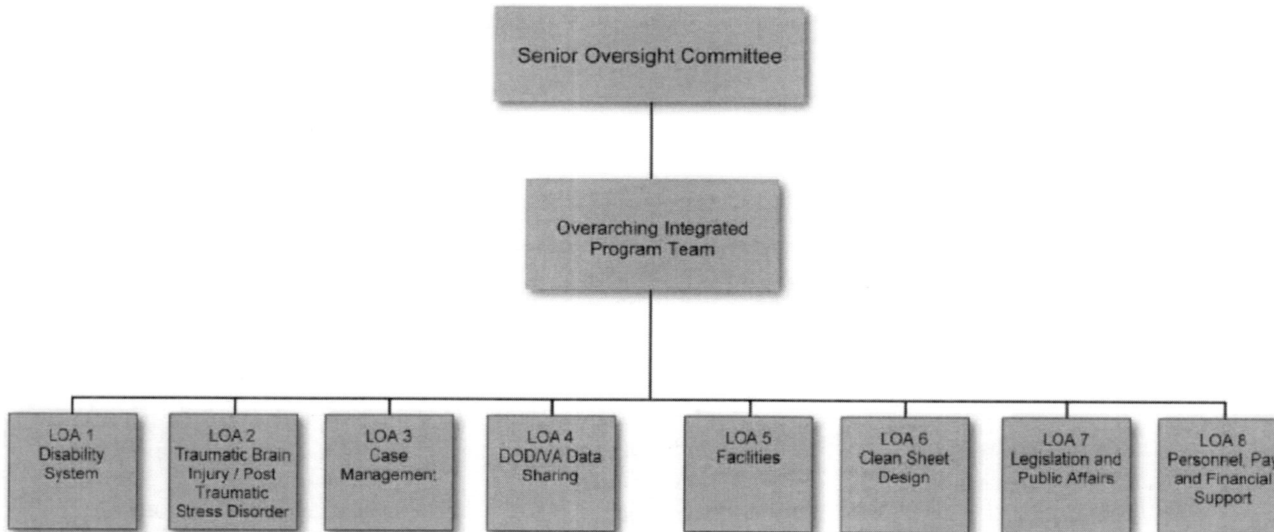

Source: Senior Oversight Committee.

Figure 2. Original Senior Oversight Committee Organizational Chart, including the Lines of Action (LOA) Workgroups.

- *LOA 7*—Legislation and Public Affairs: Responsible for addressing legal and other issues for policy development.
- *LOA 8*—Personnel, Pay, and Financial Support: Responsible for addressing compensation and benefit issues.

Some of the key efforts initiated out of the LOAs included the establishment of an integrated disability evaluation system, care coordination programs, and steps towards the electronic exchange of DOD and VA health records—a responsibility that was later assumed by the Interagency Program Office.

DOD/VA Integrated Disability Evaluation System. Through LOA 1, DOD and VA jointly began to develop and pilot IDES to improve the disability evaluation process by eliminating duplication in DOD's and VA's separate evaluation systems and expediting the receipt of VA benefits. Specifically, IDES merges DOD's and VA's separate medical exams for servicemembers into a single exam process; consolidates DOD's and VA's separate disability rating decisions into a single VA rating decision; and provides staff to perform outreach and nonclinical case management and explain VA results and processes to servicemembers. By October 2011, DOD and VA had fully deployed IDES at 139 MTFs in the United States and several other countries.

Care Coordination Programs. LOA 3 took the lead role in addressing problems with uncoordinated case management for recovering servicemembers and veterans through the establishment of two care coordination programs—the FRCP and the RCP. The FRCP was based on a recommendation from the Dole-Shalala Commission that a single individual—a recovery coordinator—would work with existing DOD and VA case managers to ensure that servicemembers had the resources needed for their care. LOA 3 designed the FRCP to assist "severely" wounded, ill, and injured OEF and OIF[18] servicemembers, veterans, and their families with access to care, services, and benefits. This population includes servicemembers and veterans who suffer from traumatic brain injuries, amputations, burns, spinal cord injuries, visual impairment, and PTSD. The program uses federal recovery coordinators to monitor and coordinate clinical services, including facilitating and coordinating medical appointments, and nonclinical services, such as providing assistance with obtaining financial benefits or special accommodations, needed by program enrollees and their families. Federal recovery coordinators, who are senior-level registered nurses and licensed clinical social workers, were intended to serve as the single point of contact among all of the case managers of DOD, VA, and other governmental and nongovernmental programs[19] that provide services directly to servicemembers and veterans. Although the FRCP was designed as a joint program, it is administered by VA, and the federal recovery coordinators are VA employees.

Table 1. Military Services' Wounded Warrior Programs: Types of Services Provided

		Types of services provided		
Military services' wounded warrior program	*Clinical case management*	*Nonclinical case management*	*Care coordination*	*Career, education, and readiness*[a]
Army				
Army Warrior Care and Transition Program: Warrior Transition Units and Community-Based Warrior Transition Units[b]	•	•		•
Army Warrior Care and Transition Program: Army Wounded Warrior Program			•	•
Navy/Coast Guard				
Navy Safe Harbor Program			•	•
Air Force				
Air Force Wounded Warrior Program		•		•
Air Force Recovery Care Program			•	•
Marine Corps				
Marine Corps Wounded Warrior Regiment		•	•	•
United States Special Operations Command				
United States Special Operations Command's Care Coalition		•	•	•

Source: GAO analysis of military services' wounded warrior program information.

Notes: The characteristics listed in this table are general characteristics of each program; individual circumstances may affect the services provided by specific programs. For the purposes of this report, clinical case management services include services such as scheduling medical appointments and providing outreach education about medical conditions such as PTSD. Nonclinical case management services include services such as assisting servicemembers with financial benefits and accessing accommodations for families.

[a] Career, education, and readiness services are provided through programs such as the Warrior Athlete Reconditioning Program and DOD's Operation Warfighter Program and Education and Employment Initiative. The Warrior Athlete Reconditioning Program enhances recovery by engaging wounded, ill, and injured servicemembers in individualized physical and cognitive activities outside of traditional therapy settings. Operation Warfighter is a federal internship program for wounded, ill, and injured servicemembers that places them in supportive work settings to prepare them to return to active duty or to transition into jobs in the government or private sector. To access the Operation Warfighter Program a recovering servicemember has to be enrolled in a military service wounded warrior program. In addition, the military services' wounded warrior programs facilitate access to other programs such as the Warrior Athlete Reconditioning Program.

[b] A warrior transition unit is technically an Army brigade, battalion, or company that provides command and control, administrative support, primary care and case management and other services to support soldiers and their families during recovery, rehabilitation, and transition back to active duty or to civilian life. For the purposes of this report, we are categorizing it as a wounded warrior program.

LOA 3 subsequently developed the RCP in response to a requirement in the NDAA 2008. The RCP is a DOD-specific program that uses recovery care coordinators to coordinate nonclinical services and resources for "seriously" wounded, ill, and injured servicemembers who may return to active duty, unlike those categorized as "severely" wounded, ill, and injured, who are not likely to return to duty and would be served by the FRCP. The military services were responsible for separately implementing the RCP through each of their existing wounded warrior programs as a means of providing care coordination services to program enrollees.

Electronic Sharing of Health Records. LOA 4 was focused on addressing issues related to the electronic exchange of DOD and VA health records. However, this effort was superseded by the NDAA 2008,[20] which required the establishment of the Interagency Program Office to serve as a single point of accountability for both departments in the development and implementation of interoperable electronic health records.[21] Although DOD and VA retained the responsibility for the development and management of the information technology systems, the Interagency Program Office was responsible for ensuring the implementation of an electronic health records system or capabilities that allowed for the complete sharing of health care information for the provision of clinical care. In October 2011, the Interagency Program Office also became accountable for DOD's and VA's work on developing an integrated electronic health records system that both departments would use for their beneficiaries.

Additional Efforts by DOD and VA to Address Problems Facing Recovering Servicemembers and Veterans

In addition to the Senior Oversight Committee's efforts, DOD, its military services, and VA developed or modified a number of programs and initiatives to assist recovering servicemembers and veterans in navigating the recovery care continuum.

Military Services' Wounded Warrior Programs. The military services' wounded warrior programs were established to assist recovering servicemembers[22] during their recovery, rehabilitation, and initial reintegration back to active duty or to civilian life.

Most of these programs provide nonclinical case management services to the recovering servicemembers; that is, they help to resolve issues related to finances, benefits and compensation, administrative and personnel paperwork, housing, and transportation. In addition, the wounded warrior programs serve as the central point of access to other types of services or resources that support recovering servicemembers, such as clinical case management, care coordination, and career, education, and readiness services. (See table 1.) If a wounded warrior program does not directly provide a service or resource, it can facilitate servicemembers' access to that service or resource. Although the wounded warrior programs were intended mainly to provide services to recovering servicemembers, all but one of the programs continue to assist individuals after they have transitioned to veteran status.

VA Transition Programs. VA's Liaison for Healthcare Program and its OEF/OIF/OND Care Management Program assist recovering servicemembers with transitioning from DOD's to VA's health care system. As of August 2012, the Liaison for Healthcare Program employed 33 liaisons at 18 MTFs nationwide.[23] After a DOD or VA treatment team determines that a recovering servicemember is medically ready to transition to a VAMC, a VA liaison facilitates the transfer from an MTF to a VAMC closest to their homes or to the most appropriate locations for the specialized services their medical condition requires. VA liaisons follow recovering servicemembers as they enter the VA health care system, ensuring that their first VA appointments are scheduled. Thereafter, the VA OEF/OIF/OND Care Management Program team assigned to each recovering individual coordinates the individual's care at the VAMC and provides ongoing follow-up.[24] Each VAMC has an OEF/OIF/OND Care Management Program team in place to coordinate patient care activities.

DOD AND VA HAVE NOT FULLY RESOLVED PERSISTENT PROBLEMS WITH CASE MANAGEMENT AND CARE COORDINATION, DISABILITY EVALUATION SYSTEMS, AND ELECTRONIC SHARING OF HEALTH RECORDS

Recovering Servicemembers and Veterans Do Not Always Have Access to the Case Management and Care Coordination Programs Designed to Assist Them

Recovering servicemembers' access to case management and care coordination programs has been impeded by two main factors—(1) the limited ability to identify and refer those servicemembers who could benefit from enrollment in the programs along with officials' reluctance to refer them, and (2) variations in eligibility criteria among the military services' wounded warrior programs, resulting in access disparities for similarly situated recovering servicemembers.[25]

Recovering Servicemembers Are Not Always Identified and Referred to Programs That May Benefit Them

We found that referrals may be lacking or delayed (1) from military service unit commanders to wounded warrior programs; (2) from wounded warrior programs to the FRCP; and (3) for certain groups of servicemembers, such as those with "invisible injuries" as well as members of the National Guard and Reserve.

Referral to the military services' wounded warrior programs. The military services' wounded warrior programs primarily use referrals to identify recovering servicemembers that might be eligible for enrollment. However, we found that the methods for referral, which include casualty reports and direct referrals, are imprecise, such that all servicemembers who could benefit from being enrolled in these programs are not necessarily identified and referred.

Officials from three wounded warrior programs told us that casualty reports are the primary method for receiving referrals.[26] Casualty reports are initial alerts to military personnel, including wounded warrior program officials, that a servicemember has been injured. These reports can be initiated by unit commands or other military personnel as a method of referral to the wounded warrior programs. However, wounded warrior program officials from four wounded warrior programs told us that casualty reports are not created after every injury or may be created late in a servicemember's recovery. In particular, some of these officials said that military service unit command staff may delay or not create casualty reports for servicemembers not injured in combat, such as for injuries that occur stateside or while on leave, because servicemembers' units may not find out about such incidents immediately.

According to wounded warrior program officials, referrals to wounded warrior programs also can be made directly from unit command staff and other sources, including staff at the MTF where a recovering servicemember is receiving treatment or through self-referrals. referrals also may not be made in a timely manner. Specifically, unit command staff may not refer potentially eligible servicemembers to wounded warrior programs because either they want to "take care of their own" or because they are not well informed about the programs and the services they provide, according to wounded warrior program officials. For example, a wounded warrior program official told us that he identified a servicemember who had sustained a gunshot wound to the head but was still assigned to his combat unit. This official explained that even though the servicemember was receiving treatment, he could have benefited from being enrolled in the wounded warrior program because of the additional assistance it provides, including nonclinical case management and care coordination services. Additionally, several recovering servicemembers told us that they encountered difficulties in their recovery as a result of staying in their units and not being referred to a wounded warrior program earlier. For example, a recovering servicemember told us that despite having been recently discharged from a hospital for arm injuries, he was required to operate a floor buffing machine in his unit, which was difficult for him as a result of his injuries. He did not receive rehabilitative treatment for his injuries until he was assigned to a wounded warrior program. Furthermore, we found that most of the military services' wounded warrior programs do not always track the number of referrals to their programs, including data on whether or not servicemembers referred to the programs were actually enrolled. (See table 14 in app. I for additional information about referral data.) Without this information, it is not clear whether all those who could benefit from a wounded warrior program are being enrolled.

Referral to the FRCP. In addition to problems with referrals to wounded warrior programs, wounded warrior program officials sometimes delay or fail to make referrals of potentially eligible servicemembers to the FRCP, which coordinates care across the departments and throughout the recovery care continuum. As we have previously reported, the FRCP relies predominantly on referrals from other sources, including wounded warrior program officials and clinical treatment teams, because it does not have a systematic way to identify potential enrollees.[28] Referrals to the FRCP are important because federal recovery coordinators are intended to provide continuity of care throughout servicemembers' recovery, starting with their initial treatment at an MTF and throughout the recovery care continuum. They can also assist in facilitating recovering servicemembers' access to VA services and benefits while servicemembers are still on active duty, according to VA officials.[29] However, we found that officials from wounded warrior programs view the jointly created and established FRCP as a VA program and, therefore, delay their referrals until it is certain that the servicemember will become a veteran.

Referrals for certain servicemember populations. We found that certain servicemember populations may be at greater risk for not being identified for DOD and VA case management and care coordination programs.

Specifically, according to wounded warrior program officials, servicemembers who have undiagnosed, "invisible" wounds, such as PTSD and TBI, may be at greater risk of not being referred to a wounded warrior program or the FRCP until it becomes apparent that the servicemember cannot be deployed. For example, a servicemember told us that although he was experiencing anxiety every time he put on his uniform, it was not until he had a severe anxiety attack, as a result of his PTSD, that he was hospitalized and then referred to a wounded warrior program. According to officials representing military advocacy organizations, National Guard and Reserve servicemembers may be particularly reluctant to identify injuries and illnesses because they are eager to return home and do not want to be delayed at the installation for an evaluation of any conditions they may have. However, these officials said that when these servicemembers have been deactivated and problems manifest themselves later on, they may experience difficulties establishing that their injuries or illnesses are a result of their service in the military, which could make it difficult for them to access services and programs provided by DOD and VA.

Recovering Servicemembers' Access to the Military Services' Wounded Warrior Programs Is Likely to Be Inequitable Due to Variations in Their Eligibility Criteria

Because of variations in eligibility criteria among the military services' wounded warrior programs, DOD cannot assure that similarly situated servicemembers have equitable access to these programs, leading to disparities in the level of assistance provided across the military services. (See table 2.) For example, servicemembers can only be eligible for the Air Force Wounded Warrior Program if they have a combat-related injury or illness, whereas servicemembers with combat or non-combat-related injuries or illnesses can be eligible for the Army's Warrior Transition Units.

Table 2. Eligibility Criteria for Military Services' Wounded Warrior Programs

Military services' wounded warrior program	Eligibility criteria
Army	
Army Warrior Care and Transition Program: Warrior Transition Units and Community-Based Warrior Transition Units	Serves servicemembers who require at least 6 months of rehabilitative care and complex medical management[a]
Army Warrior Care and Transition Program: Army Wounded Warrior Program	Serves "severely" wounded, ill, and injured servicemembers in the warrior transition units who have, or are expected to receive, a physical evaluation disability rating[b] of 30 percent or greater in one or more specific categories or a combined rating of 50 percent or greater for conditions that are combat-related
Navy/Coast Guard	
Navy Safe Harbor Program	Serves "seriously" wounded, ill, and injured sailors and coast guardsmen not likely to return to duty in 180 days and likely to be medically retired, as well as high-risk wounded, ill, and injured sailors that have less serious health concerns
Air Force	
Air Force Wounded Warrior Program	Serves servicemembers with a combat-related injury or illness that requires long-term care[c] as well as examinations to determine fitness for

Military services' wounded warrior program	Eligibility criteria
	duty
Air Force Recovery Care Program	Serves all servicemembers who are "seriously" [d] ill and injured either in a combat-related incident or in a non-combat-related incident
Marine Corps	
Marine Corps Wounded Warrior Regiment	Serves wounded, ill, and injured servicemembers who require more than 90 days of medical treatment or rehabilitation. A recovering servicemember also may be assigned to the Wounded Warrior Regiment when: • the unit command cannot support transportation requirements to the military treatment facility, • the Marine cannot serve a function in the unit command due to his/her injuries or illness, or • the Marine has three or more medical appointments per week.
United States Special Operations Command	
United States Special Operations Command's Care Coalition	Assists Special Forces servicemembers who are • wounded, injured, or ill evacuated from a combat area; • wounded, injured, or ill returned to duty or redeployed; or • injured or ill whose injury or illness is not combat-related.

Source: GAO analysis of military services' wounded warrior program information.

[a] Reservists in need of definitive medical treatment for conditions caused or aggravated while on active duty or training status are also eligible.

[b] After medical examinations are conducted to determine a servicemember's ability to continue to serve in the military, decisions are made about the servicemember's fitness for duty and about a servicemember's disability rating, which determines the DOD and VA benefits he or she can receive.

[c] According to an Air Force Wounded Warrior Program official, the program does not define long-term care or provide criteria related to the time needed for recovery.

[d] According to an Air Force Recovery Care Program official, a servicemember is designated as "seriously' ill or injured on the basis of a medical diagnosis made by Air Force medical staff when referred to the program; the program does not make this designation.

As a result of these differences in eligibility criteria, recovering servicemembers in one military service may qualify for entry in their wounded warrior program while similarly situated servicemembers in another military service do not have access to their program. Consequently, according to wounded warrior program officials, some recovering servicemembers do not have access to services that would otherwise be available to them, including the RCP and Operation Warfighter.[30] Additionally, because wounded warrior programs facilitate access to other programs and services, including the VA Liaison for Healthcare Program and the Warrior Athlete Reconditioning Program,[31] not being eligible for a particular wounded warrior program could preclude a servicemember from receiving the services of these other programs.[32] Military coalition officials who advocate for recovering servicemembers and their families told us the lack of standardization across similar programs, such as the military services' wounded warrior programs, is one of the main reasons recovering servicemembers "fall through the cracks" or do not get the services that they need when they are navigating the recovery care continuum.

DOD is aware of inconsistencies in eligibility criteria among the military services' wounded warrior programs and the potential for disparities in the provision of services and assistance that may result. DOD has not taken action to correct this, however, despite the identification of this issue as a potential problem for recovering servicemembers by a congressionally mandated DOD task force. Specifically, in its 2011 annual report to congressional committees, the Recovering Warrior Task Force noted that as a result of differences in eligibility criteria among the military services, certain subpopulations of recovering servicemembers may be at a disadvantage.[33] In response to this report, DOD stated that although there are no DOD-wide criteria for entry into wounded warrior programs, the individual military services already have policies in place as a result of the flexibility given to them by DOD.

Delays in DOD's and VA's Integrated Disability Evaluation System Persist, Limiting Recovering Servicemembers' Ability to Plan for Their Future

Although IDES provides improved timeliness over the separate DOD and VA disability evaluation systems, processing times have continued to increase since its implementation in November 2007, resulting in frustration and uncertainty for servicemembers going through the process. In a May 2012 hearing,[34] we testified that the average number of days for servicemembers to complete the IDES process and receive VA benefits increased from 283 in fiscal year 2008 to 394 in fiscal year 2011 for active duty cases (compared to the goal of 295 days) and from 297 to 420 for reserve cases, respectively (compared to the goal of 305 days).[35]

While there are many reasons for increases in processing times,[36] recovering servicemembers and wounded warrior program officials told us that extended timelines in the IDES process and the lack of a firm completion date limits recovering servicemembers' ability to plan for their future. Several recovering servicemembers said that not being given a timeframe for completion of the IDES process is frustrating, particularly when their own providers are unable to obtain additional information on the status of their case. For example, a servicemember told us that after going through the IDES process, receiving a rating, and filing an appeal over a year ago, he still did not know the status of his case, negatively affecting his ability to plan for his future. Similarly, a wounded warrior program official also told us that her program has had several servicemembers lose job opportunities because they applied for positions thinking that they would be through the IDES process by a certain date, but when that date was pushed back, the employers rescinded their offers.

Wounded warrior program officials from some of the sites we visited told us that extended waiting periods resulting from the disability process also may lead to some recovering servicemembers engaging in negative behavior, including drug use. Wounded warrior program officials told us that after waiting for so long in the wounded warrior barracks due to the lengthy disability process, servicemembers can get depressed, resist or just stop going to medical appointments, and stop working on their recovery. Similarly, the DOD Inspector General has reported that lengthy IDES processing times has contributed to a negative and even counterproductive environment, which was not conducive to servicemembers' recovery and transition.[37] To prevent these problems, we found that two wounded warrior programs require recovering servicemembers to participate in programs such as the Warrior Athlete Reconditioning Program and Operation Warfighter. A recovering servicemember told us that soon after being assigned to the wounded warrior program, he was referred to the Warrior Athlete Reconditioning Program, which gave him something to do other than "sitting around." Another recovering servicemember told us that the Warrior Athlete Reconditioning Program is an effective motivator for recovery.

Conversely, the servicemembers could take actions that may impact their own processing times in IDES and, therefore, their length of stay in a wounded warrior program. We found that some servicemembers may appeal their disability decisions to prolong their own recovery and transition out of the military. According to wounded warrior program officials from some of the sites we visited, some servicemembers resist their transfer out of the wounded warrior program and the military because they want to continue to take advantage of the opportunities and services available to them, including the financial security of a regular paycheck. For example, a wounded warrior program official and a VA official told us that some servicemembers will purposefully miss appointments to delay the IDES process because they feel that they are not ready to leave the program.

DOD and VA Have Yet to Develop Sufficient Capability to Electronically Share Health Records, Potentially Delaying Servicemembers' Receipt of Coordinated Care and Benefits

The departments have not yet developed sufficient capability to electronically share servicemembers' and veterans' complete health records, which can delay the receipt of care and benefits for recovering servicemembers and veterans. As we have previously reported, for over a decade DOD and VA have undertaken several efforts to improve the ability of their information technology systems to electronically share health records.[38] For example, the Federal Health Information Exchange, which was started in 2001 and completed in 2004, allows DOD to electronically transfer servicemembers' health information to VA when they leave active duty. In addition, the departments' Bidirectional Health Information Exchange was established in 2004 to allow clinicians in both departments to view limited health information on patients who receive care from both departments. More recently, the departments have undertaken two new joint initiatives, the Virtual Lifetime Electronic Record and an integrated electronic health records system, in an effort to increase electronic health record interoperability and modernize their systems.

We found that although DOD and VA care providers were expected to have access to some electronic health record information across the departments, the DOD and VA care providers that we spoke to still did not have the ability to electronically share complete health records for recovering servicemembers who were transferring between DOD's and VA's health care systems, and therefore they had to use other methods.

For example, wounded warrior program and VA officials told us that they had to resort to copying and faxing recovering servicemembers' health records to VAMC staff in preparation for a servicemember's transition from DOD's to VA's health care system because there was not an automatic, electronic way to transfer them. In addition to copying and faxing health records, according to VA officials we spoke with, DOD and VA staff may hold a video-teleconference between the transferring MTF and receiving VA health care facilities to exchange information.

In addition, wounded warrior program and VA officials who help servicemembers transition from DOD to VA told us that they only share with VA facilities the health records necessary for the treatment of a recovering servicemember's current condition. As a result, servicemembers' and veterans' complete health records are not always shared between departments when transferring facilities, and ultimately, the responsibility to collect and provide a complete health record to the VA facility can fall on the recovering servicemember and veteran.[39] A VA official told us that this process can be complicated because DOD separately maintains servicemembers' inpatient, outpatient, and behavioral health records and does not have a single database that can identify all of the medical facilities where a servicemember received treatment. Further, according to VA and DOD officials, delaying the collection and assembly of a servicemember's complete medical history until the start of the disability process could result in servicemembers having to be reexamined when they are demobilized, needing to establish that their injuries were connected to their time in the military, thus possibly delaying a servicemember's or veteran's receipt of VA benefits.

Both departments have needed to create programs and provide staff to assist recovering servicemembers during their transition from a DOD MTF to a VAMC. For example, VA Liaisons and DOD nurse case managers help recovering servicemembers transition from DOD to VA by assembling their health records and sharing them with the VAMC where the servicemember will be receiving treatment. According to DOD and VA staff that assist servicemembers in their transition from one system to another, DOD nurse case managers at installations that do not have VA Liaisons do not always have the same knowledge of VA services and benefits, and may not be informed of the appropriate referral methods or contacts used by VA Liaisons to provide a servicemember with a seamless transition to a VAMC. A DOD official told us that at locations where the VA Liaison program is not available, the transition process for recovering servicemembers from DOD to VA is more difficult.

This official understood how to properly transfer servicemembers' records from the DOD facility to the receiving VA facility only because of past VA experience.

DOD AND VA HAVE NOT FULLY RESOLVED LONG-STANDING PROBLEMS DUE TO DEFICIENCIES IN LEADERSHIP AND OVERSIGHT, RESOURCES, AND COLLABORATION

Lack of Leadership and Oversight Has Limited DOD's and VA's Ability to Effectively Manage Programs for Recovering Servicemembers and Veterans

The lack of leadership and program oversight has limited DOD's and VA's ability to effectively manage programs created to serve recovering servicemembers and veterans. Two bodies established to oversee these programs, the Senior Oversight Committee and the Office of Wounded Warrior Care and Transition Policy (WWCTP),[40] lacked consistent leadership attention and oversight capabilities. In addition, DOD does not have a central office that oversees or collects common data on the military services' wounded warrior programs.

Strength of Senior Oversight Committee Leadership Waned

Before the Senior Oversight Committee was consolidated into the Joint Executive Council[41] in early 2012, it had already lost many of the characteristics that had made it a strong decision making and oversight body for the programs and initiatives created to assist recovering servicemembers and veterans. What had originally made it strong were

- high-level leadership participation without substitution of lower-ranking officials,
- rapid policy development and quick decision making, and
- rigorous monitoring to hold the military services and the two departments accountable for needed actions.

Sustaining the Senior Oversight Committee's original momentum over time became difficult, and its waning influence and effectiveness became evident in a number of ways:

- Starting in December 2008, the Senior Oversight Committee experienced leadership changes, including the departure of its cochairs, the Deputy Secretaries,[42] as well as turnover in some of its key staff. According to a former Senior Oversight Committee executive, the personal commitment and strong relationship between the Deputy Secretaries who initially cochaired the Senior Oversight Committee served as a unifying and confidence building force that was not replicated by subsequent leadership, while leadership turnover in the DOD offices supporting the Senior Oversight Committee negatively impacted its ability to function effectively.
- As we have previously reported, the Senior Oversight Committee also began to encounter challenges when DOD "disrupted the unity of command" by changing the organizational structure of the committee and realigning and incorporating the committee's staff and responsibilities into existing or newly created DOD and VA offices, such as WWCTP.[43] Officials formerly involved with the committee told us that the new staffing arrangement did not adequately support the committee's efforts, and VA did not provide full-time staff members to support the committee, as it had in the past. Later in October 2008, VA established the Office of VA/DOD Collaboration Services, and VA supported Senior Oversight Committee efforts, along with broader collaboration efforts, through this separate office.
- The committee began meeting less frequently. For example, in contrast to weekly meetings held during its initial year of operation, in fiscal year 2011, the committee met less than 11 hours in total.
- Top DOD leadership no longer consistently attended Senior Oversight Committee meetings. According to a former Senior Oversight Committee official, the second Deputy Secretary of Defense to cochair the committee sent the Deputy Undersecretary of Defense for Personnel and Readiness to represent DOD in his place.
- The Senior Oversight Committee no longer made relatively quick decisions. According to former Senior Oversight Committee executive and support staff, frequent substitutions by lower-ranking officials at Senior Oversight Committee meetings no longer allowed

for quick decision making and transformed Senior Oversight Committee meetings into informational briefings.

- The Senior Oversight Committee no longer tracked or monitored progress of its policy initiatives or assigned tasks. According to a former LOA cochair and a cognizant support staff member, by 2011 the Senior Oversight Committee was no longer routinely using a tracking mechanism to hold the departments accountable for completing appointed tasks. Later that year, the Recovering Warrior Task Force reported that the Senior Oversight Committee no longer had a formal mechanism for assessing the status of the committee's initiatives and goals, leaving no way to determine whether initiatives or goals had been partially or fully implemented or met.

In its September 2011 report, the Recovering Warrior Task Force recommended combining the Senior Oversight Committee and Joint Executive Council to improve effectiveness and reduce redundancies as both entities had similar membership and operating structures. In January 2012, the Joint Executive Council cochairs agreed to consolidate the two groups. The Senior Oversight Committee's working groups for care coordination and the integrated disability evaluation system were realigned within the Joint Executive Council, and a Wounded, Ill, and Injured Council was established under the Joint Executive Council to oversee emerging issues for recovering servicemembers and veterans.

Whether the Joint Executive Council can effectively address the issues once managed by the Senior Oversight Committee has yet to be seen. Several DOD and VA officials expressed concern to us about the ability of the Joint Executive Council to focus on rapid, short-term policy decision making rather than the longer-term strategic planning role that it has traditionally played. For example, according to a DOD official, historically, the Joint Executive Council has not been able to drive policy decision making, and therefore, issues that should have been decided by the Joint Executive Council were taken directly to the Secretaries for resolution, raising doubts about the ability of the Joint Executive Council to function effectively. A former Senior Oversight Committee executive noted that the Joint Executive Council cochairs are not of equivalent rank, another challenge that may serve as a barrier to the council's ability to make decisions and drive policy changes. Specifically, the VA cochair is the Deputy Secretary, who has control over all relevant offices within VA, while the DOD cochair is the Deputy Undersecretary of Defense for Personnel and Readiness, whose responsibilities include establishing health and benefit policies affecting recovering servicemembers and directing the military services to comply with such policies but lacks authority in enforcing the military services' implementation of these policies. The Recovering Warrior Task Force also cited concerns about the rank of the DOD cochair of the Joint Executive Council, stating that a higher level of leadership is needed to sustain departmental attention on key initiatives such as IDES and electronic health records.[44] Furthermore, as of August 2012, DOD officials told us that the Joint Executive Council is operating under the original procedures that were in place prior to the entities merging. As a result, it is unclear at this time how the Joint Executive Council will provide oversight and accountability for issues once addressed by the Senior Oversight Committee.

WWCTP Lacks Authority and Leadership to Provide Oversight for Care Coordination

In 2008, WWCTP became responsible for overseeing the RCP among other programs that provide assistance to recovering servicemembers. However, WWCTP's ability to oversee the RCP, including its ability to monitor program performance and ensure compliance with DOD policy, is limited by its lack of operational authority, such as budget and tasking authority, over the military services that implement the program. According to WWCTP officials, this lack of operational authority challenges WWCTP's ability to direct the military services on their implementation of the program. For example, although WWCTP has been responsible for RCP oversight since 2008, the office was not able to collect basic program data, such as monthly enrollment numbers, on a consistent basis until October 2011. According to a WWCTP official, although WWCTP requested monthly data submissions from the military services, the information was provided on an ad hoc basis; sometimes the services would submit it, and other times they would not. Data-collection efforts still remain a challenge for WWCTP. For example, the Army's Wounded Warrior Program, which serves as the Army's care coordination program, only agrees to share partial data with WWCTP, arguing that the Army is only obligated to share data on servicemembers served by WWCTP-contracted personnel.

Getting the military services to implement consistent care coordination policies also poses a challenge for WWCTP. WWCTP officials said that while WWCTP can develop policy to guide the military services, the military services may interpret that policy and implement their programs differently. Consequently, some DOD officials assert that the military services have not consistently implemented the RCP in accordance with DOD policy—an observation that is shared by the Recovering Warrior Task Force.[45] DOD policy requires that care coordination should be provided to those who are "seriously" and "severely" wounded, ill, and injured, but the Army only provides care coordination to recovering servicemembers who are "severely" wounded, ill, and injured.[46] As a result, some servicemembers who could benefit from having someone coordinate their care and benefits as they navigate the recovery care continuum do not have access to those services.

Some WWCTP officials with whom we spoke expressed the view that the military services have been inconsistent in their cooperation with WWCTP, with cooperation being better on issues that represent priorities of top leadership. Specifically, WWCTP officials told us that top DOD leadership has not been pressured to resolve lingering care coordination issues as much as other more visible issues, such as IDES and electronic medical record interoperability problems confronting the departments. Consequently, WWCTP officials said that the military services cooperate with WWCTP's efforts to oversee IDES and to monitor whether the military services achieve their goals for timely completion of the IDES process. Although these goals have not consistently been achieved,[47] the officials told us that military service cooperation has not been an impediment to overseeing IDES as it has been for overseeing care coordination. Conversely, the military services have not been as inclined to cooperate with WWCTP on its oversight of the RCP relative to these other issues.

In addition to limited operational authority over the military services, turnover in leadership and other staffing changes have also limited WWCTP's ability to provide consistent direction and oversight for the RCP, according to WWCTP officials. Specifically:

- Three different DOD officials have led WWCTP since its inception in 2008. According to WWCTP staff, each of these officials had different visions and priorities for the office, which led to disruptions in RCP oversight. For example, a major oversight initiative—to collect satisfaction survey data across the RCP—was abandoned when a new official was appointed. In addition, the RCP has been led by three different directors, with the most recent director leaving in June 2012.
- In September through December 2011, WWCTP's contracted staffing was temporarily reduced by 70 percent when a contract expired and was not immediately renewed, according to DOD. Staff reductions

primarily impacted WWCTP's ability to oversee the RCP, since many RCP support staff members were lost. For example, according to a WWCTP official, the office was no longer able to make monitoring visits to the RCP program sites. However, in July 2012 a contract was awarded that allowed WWCTP to engage additional staff to support the RCP, according to a WWCTP official.

- In June 2012, DOD changed the name of the WWCTP office to the Office of Warrior Care Policy and moved it under the Assistant Secretary of Defense for Health Affairs. According to a DOD official, the change was made as part of a realignment of DOD's organizational structure in response to statutory requirements.[48] An official in Health Affairs said that the move will be beneficial because it will provide greater access to resources, including human resources and information technology, among others. However, it is too early to determine the full effect of this change.

Wounded Warrior Programs Lack Central Oversight

There is currently no central office or authority that oversees or collects common data on the military services' wounded warrior programs, preventing DOD from both assessing how well the programs are working across the department and leveraging the strengths of each program by sharing proven best practices across the military services.

Each of the military service Secretaries created their own wounded warrior programs to meet their military service's unique needs. Because each service developed its own policy to govern its wounded warrior programs and no central, unified DOD policy exists to govern these programs, no central DOD office—such as WWCTP—may direct how these programs operate. This lack of central oversight over the wounded warrior programs has been one of the main reasons for the large discrepancies between these programs. The 2011 Recovering Warrior Task Force report recommended that the Secretary of Defense enforce the existing policy guidance regarding the Army's and Marines' wounded warrior transition units' entrance criteria. However, in its response to this recommendation, DOD supported the military service Secretaries' discretion in establishing their own policies in this regard, saying that there is no central DOD policy on the establishment of transition units and entrance criteria, and that the policies were established by the Secretaries for their specific populations.

While no common data are collected on the performance of wounded warrior programs across the military services, each individual program has initiated internal efforts to collect and analyze performance data. The type and quality of data vary by program, however. For example, the largest of the wounded warrior programs, the Army Warrior Care and Transition Program, has collected wounded warrior program performance survey data on a continuous basis since March 2007 and has developed outcome measures to determine the impact of its services.

Table 3. Military Services' Wounded Warrior Program Efforts to Measure Program Performance

Military services' wounded warrior program	Satisfaction surveys: Measures customer satisfaction with program	Performance metrics: Measures whether program meets target output goals	Outcome measures: Measures whether program achieves desired impact
Army			
Army Warrior Care and Transition Program	•	•	•
Army Wounded Warrior Program	•	•	•
Navy/Coast Guard			
Navy Safe Harbor Program	•	•	
Air Force			
Air Force Wounded Warrior Program	•[a]		
Air Force Recovery Care Program	•[a]	•	
Marine Corps			
Marine Corps Wounded Warrior Regiment	•	•	•
United States Special Operations Command			
United States Special Operations Command's Care Coalition	•	•[b]	

Source: GAO analysis of interviews with military services' wounded warrior program officials and program documentation.

[a] Although the Air Force Wounded Warrior and Recovery Care Programs' initial satisfaction survey was completed in October 2011, the survey results have not been released as of August 9, 2012.

[b] The United States Special Operations Command's Care Coalition has performance metrics for its Recovery Program.

However, smaller programs, such as the Air Force Wounded Warrior Program and the United States Special Operations Command's Care Coalition have measured baseline program satisfaction levels, but they do not have additional years of survey data to monitor any changes over time. (See table 3 for information about the types of performance data collected by each of the wounded warrior programs.)

Some DOD officials with whom we spoke questioned why common measures have not been developed. For example, a DOD official in charge of wounded warrior care at an MTF suggested developing a measurement tool to determine what aspects of the programs help recovering servicemembers. Another DOD official involved with wounded warrior program performance measurement commented that it is common practice for DOD to share performance measurement practices and standard metrics across the military services. In September 2011, citing wide disparity across the military services in their implementation of wounded warrior programs and policies, the Recovering Warrior Task Force made four recommendations for creating common standards to ensure parity in the programs and services provided to recovering servicemembers across DOD.49 For example, the first recommendation called for a common nomenclature, or consistent definitions to be used in DOD policy to identify recovering servicemembers who may require and be eligible for assistance. The task force concluded that common definitions are needed to promote consistent levels of care among the military services and would better enable DOD to compare across programs and identify best practices. In its response to the task force, DOD acknowledged that some of these recommendations were valid and that DOD should take actions to address them. However, at the time of the Recovering Warrior Task Force's 2012 report, these recommendations had not been implemented, and the task force is continuing to follow DOD's efforts to implement them.50 Moreover, even if DOD decided to take some actions in this regard, it is unclear who would have responsibility for addressing them, since there is no central oversight office or authority for these programs.

Insufficient Staffing and Budget Control Have Contributed to DOD's and VA's Inability to Resolve Delays with Disability Determinations and Electronically Share Health Records

In addition to problems with leadership and oversight of care coordination and case management programs, DOD and VA have a longstanding track record of insufficient staffing to address delays in disability determinations and insufficient staffing and control over the budget to oversee the development of systems with improved capabilities for electronically sharing health records.[51]

Insufficient Staffing Contributed to Delays in Disability Determinations

Insufficient staffing across both departments has affected DOD's and VA's ability to reduce disability determination delays and meet their IDES timeliness goals. We raised concerns about staffing in 2010, when we reported that DOD and VA did not sufficiently staff many key positions in the IDES process, including DOD board liaisons, who counsel servicemembers and ensure that documentation submitted for consideration is complete and accurate, and medical evaluation board physicians, who review medical and service records to identify conditions that limit a servicemember's ability to serve in the military.[52] In 2012, we continued to report evidence of staffing shortages, including high caseloads for DOD board liaisons and VA case managers as well as insufficient numbers of physicians to write narrative summaries needed to complete the medical evaluation board stage of the IDES process in a timely manner.[53] Some recovering servicemembers told us they do not receive sufficient support from their DOD board liaisons, and that there are not enough liaisons to efficiently meet the needs of all the recovering servicemembers going through the IDES process.

Delays in the disability determination process are expected to continue. VA anticipates a much larger caseload of all disability and other benefit claims in the near future, not just those claims associated with IDES cases. Specifically, a high-level VA official told us that new laws, such as the Veterans Opportunity to Work Act,[54] will encourage all transitioning servicemembers—not just those going through the IDES process—to claim VA benefits. This official also told us that DOD and VA have a much larger problem to address as a surge of 300,000 servicemembers begin to transition into the VA system as troops return home from Iraq and Afghanistan. Without adequate planning and adequate resources, these servicemembers may experience much longer processing times in the disability benefits systems.

DOD and VA are working to address staffing challenges in some of the IDES processes that are most delayed. We have previously reported that the Army, for example, is in the midst of a major hiring initiative to increase staffing dedicated to its medical evaluation boards, which will include additional DOD board liaisons and medical evaluation board physician positions.[55] Additionally, VA officials said that the agency has added staffing to its IDES rating sites to handle the demand for preliminary disability ratings, rating reconsiderations, and final benefit decisions, which has increased the number of preliminary VA ratings completed and slightly improved processing times. But it is too early to tell the extent to which VA's efforts will continue to improve processing times.

Lack of Staffing and Budget Control Limited Progress on Electronic Health Records Sharing

The Interagency Program Office was established by law[56] to serve as a single point of accountability for joint DOD and VA efforts to implement fully interoperable electronic health record systems or capabilities, but this office was not given sufficient staffing or budget control by DOD and VA to effectively facilitate the departments' efforts. According to an Interagency Program Office official, the office was never fully staffed and was challenged by a high degree of turnover in staffing and leadership that served in a temporary or acting capacity.

The Interagency Program Office's initial charter limited its ability to exercise authority over DOD and VA. Specifically, the charter stated that control of the budget, contracts, and technical development remained wholly within the two departments' program offices. The charter conveyed no authority in these areas to the Interagency Program Office. As a former Interagency Program Office official testified in July 2011, the office lacked control of budgeting and contracting necessary to achieve its intended purpose, and without this, it could not sufficiently oversee the departments' efforts and compliance with the requirements in NDAA 2008.[57] As a result, each department continued to pursue separate strategies, rather than a unified interoperable approach, according to this former official.

The Interagency Program Office was rechartered in October 2011 and provided an expanded staff and new authorities under the charter, including control over the budget. According to Interagency Program Office officials, when hiring under the new charter is completed, the office will have a staff of 236 personnel, more than seven times the number of staff originally allotted to the office by DOD and VA.[58]

In addition, the charter provides the Interagency Program Office with the authority to lead, oversee, and manage budget and contracting for electronic health record sharing efforts.

According to Interagency Program Office officials, budget control is the essential component for overseeing progress and ensuring accountability for the departments' efforts.

With the enhanced charter, as well as plans for an expanded staff to oversee the implementation of a single joint electronic health record system, the Interagency Program Office will have more resources to draw upon and support department interoperability initiatives. However, it is still too early to determine whether this investment of resources will be sufficient to meet the office's goals for 2017.[59] For example, despite the provision of additional resources, Interagency Program Office officials told us that as of July 2012, the office is staffed at approximately 48 percent and that hiring additional staff in time to meet appointed implementation deadlines remains one of its biggest challenges.

Despite Repeated Attempts, DOD and VA Have Failed to Effectively Collaborate to Align Their Care Coordination Programs; New Efforts Are under Way

Since the inception of the RCP in 2008, the FRCP and RCP care coordination programs have conflicted with one another and with other case management programs that provide services to recovering servicemembers and veterans. Conflicting issues have arisen as to what populations they serve, the specific services each would provide, and when each program would get involved in the servicemembers' recovery process. Aligning and integrating these programs with one another— especially the FRCP with the RCP—has proven to be a major challenge for DOD and VA. While the departments are developing an interagency strategy for minimizing duplication between DOD's and VA's care coordination and case management programs, the success of this effort will depend upon achieving cooperation between the departments—which has been elusive for many years—as well as with the military services.

With the creation of the RCP, the FRCP was no longer the single point of contact with respect to servicemembers' care coordination, and early on, there were concerns and some confusion about how the FRCP and the RCP would align without creating overlapping and duplicative services. Shortly after the RCP was established, DOD sent a report to congressional committees outlining a medical category assignment process that was based on the severity of each servicemember's medical condition, along with input from the servicemember and his or her unit commander, to determine whether servicemembers would be directed to either the FRCP or to the RCP for care coordination services. In concept, the medical category assignment process would have resulted in wounded, ill, and injured servicemembers being assigned to one of three categories: "mild," "serious," or "severe." Under this approach, the FRCP would provide care coordination services for "severely" wounded, ill, and injured servicemembers and the RCP would serve those who were "seriously" wounded, ill, and injured. (See app. II for additional information on the intended medical category assignment process for DOD and VA care coordination programs.)

Despite DOD's attempt to define the populations served by the FRCP and the RCP, neither the military services' wounded warrior programs, which implement the RCP, nor VA, which administers the FRCP, implemented DOD's assignment process. Instead, these programs expanded their enrollment to include both "seriously" and "severely" recovering servicemembers and veterans, which resulted in both programs serving the same populations, thereby setting up the likelihood of overlap and duplication of services. As we have previously reported, this duplication issue is compounded by the numerous other programs that also provide services to recovering servicemembers and veterans and have overlapping roles as well. It is not uncommon for recovering servicemembers to be enrolled in more than one case management or care coordination program and end up with multiple care coordinators and case managers—each of whom develop different care plans for the same servicemember. The care plans may even conflict with one another, which could conceivably adversely affect the servicemember's recovery process. In fact, in the course of previous work, we found instances where inadequate information exchange and poor coordination between these programs resulted not only in duplication of effort and overlap of services, but also confusion and frustration for servicemembers and their families.[60] In addition, DOD and VA officials acknowledge that the multiplicity of care coordination and case management programs causes confusion even among members of care coordination teams. In October 2011, we recommended that the Secretaries of Defense and Veterans Affairs direct the Senior Oversight Committee to expeditiously develop and implement a plan to strengthen functional integration across all DOD and VA care coordination and case management programs to reduce redundancy and overlap.

Although DOD and VA have not yet aligned care coordination policy for the FRCP and RCP, we have found indications that care coordinators and case managers at some locations have been cooperating to some degree and trying to work more closely with one another. In the course of our visits to 11 DOD and VA facilities during this review, we found that care coordinators and case managers in many locations had attempted—with some success—to clarify their roles and to limit the degree of overlap and duplication in the services they provide to recovering servicemembers and veterans. However, such local attempts to improve the degree of cooperation and coordination among the programs are not systemic and depend on individual personalities and circumstances. They may not be sustainable without agreement by DOD and VA and the alignment of policy governing case management and care coordination programs.

Another critical issue on which DOD and VA have disagreed pertains to the stage in a servicemember's recovery when the FRCP should get involved in the coordination of services. Because the FRCP depends on referrals from other programs as a basis for becoming involved with recovering servicemembers, this can be a significant issue. Currently, neither DOD nor VA policy clearly defines when referrals are to be made; consequently, most wounded warrior programs delay referrals to the FRCP until it becomes clear that the servicemember will be separated from the military. Senior DOD officials stated that wounded warrior program officials justify this practice on the basis that referring a recently wounded servicemember to the FRCP—a VA-operated program—sends a negative message to a recovering servicemember that his or her military career has ended, even though the FRCP was designed as a joint program. Additionally, the belief among the military that they should "take care of their own," contributes to the reluctance to involve the FRCP. On their part, VA maintains that its point of engagement should be in the early stage of medical treatment to build rapport and trust and to begin coordinating the services needed by severely wounded servicemembers.

Despite multiple efforts over the last several years to align their care coordination and case management programs, DOD and VA have failed to implement lasting measures to resolve underlying problems concerning the aligning of roles and responsibilities of the FRCP, RCP, and case management programs. Previous attempts include the following:

- *December 2010.* The Senior Oversight Committee directed its case management work group to perform a feasibility study of recommendations on the governance, roles, and mission of DOD and VA care coordination. However, no action was taken by the committee and care coordination was subsequently removed from the Senior Oversight Committee's agenda as other issues were given higher priority.

- *March 2011.* WWCTP sponsored a joint summit that included officials from VA and the military services to review DOD and VA care coordination issues. Although this collaboration resulted in the development of five recommendations related to care coordination, no agreement was reached by the departments to jointly implement them. A DOD participant told us that VA did not agree with the recommendations, and a VA official involved in the summit concurred, alleging that the recommendations appeared to suggest eliminating overlap and duplication between the FRCP and RCP by ending the FRCP.
- *May 2011.* Concerned with overlap and duplication between the DOD and VA care coordination programs, the House Committee on Veterans Affairs, Subcommittee on Health directed the Deputy Secretaries of DOD and VA to provide an analysis of how the FRCP and RCP could be integrated under a "single umbrella" by June 20, 2011. In the absence of such a response, the subcommittee scheduled a congressional hearing and requested that options for addressing this issue be presented. Following the notification of the hearing, the departments developed a joint letter and submitted it to the subcommittee in September 2011. This letter, however, did not identify or outline options for aligning the FRCP and the RCP. In a hearing held by the subcommittee in early October 2011, neither VA nor DOD outlined definitive plans to address this issue.
- *September 2011.* The Recovering Warrior Task Force issued the first of four annual reports that included 21 recommendations, including a recommendation that the roles of care coordinators be clarified. In DOD's official response to congressional committees, the Under Secretary of Defense stated that the department would implement the Recovering Warrior Task Force's recommendations. However, a Recovering Warrior Task Force member stated that the Recovering Warrior Task Force concluded that in most cases DOD has not made significant changes to its programs to achieve the outcomes intended by the recommendations. In August 2012, the Recovering Warrior Task Force reported that DOD has fully implemented only 2 of the 21 recommendations.61 However, a DOD official whose office is responsible for coordinating DOD's responses to the Recovering Warrior Task Force's recommendations stated that DOD is in the process of addressing several more of the 2011 Recovering Warrior Task Force recommendations.

- *October 2011–April 2012.* VA declined DOD's requests to discuss care coordination and case management policy issues during this period, according to DOD and VA senior officials, because VA had established its own task force to conduct an internal review of its care coordination and case management activities, including the FRCP.62 After completing its initial assessment, VA briefed WWCTP officials on the process it was using to review its care coordination and case management activities, but chose not to discuss realignment of the FRCP and RCP at that time, according to DOD officials who attended this briefing. Instead, the VA Chief of Staff said that he approached the Army's Warrior Transition Command—which has the largest number of recovering servicemembers—to propose developing guidelines for better integrating Army's wounded warrior program with the FRCP, including identifying when the Army's wounded warrior programs should refer a recovering servicemember to the FRCP, and replacing multiple care coordination plans with a single, comprehensive planning document. However, a high-level DOD official criticized this initiative as a tactic to minimize central input from the Office of the Secretary of Defense and pointed out that this effort would result in an agreement with only a single military branch. In contrast, VA's Chief of Staff told us that VA took this approach in the hope that if an agreement could be reached with Army, the other military branches would follow suit.

More recently, in May 2012, VA and DOD developed a new task force, the VA/DOD Warrior Care and Coordination Task Force, which represents an effort to comprehensively address problems caused by the lack of integration between DOD's and VA's care coordination and case management programs. The task force has developed recommendations that are intended to achieve a coordinated, interdepartmental approach to care coordination and case management programs, according to a task force official. On August 10, 2012, the task force presented the following recommendations to the Joint Executive Council for its consideration:

- establish and charter an interagency governance structure responsible for coordinating VA and DOD policy,
- establish and charter an interagency care coordination community of practice,[63]

- align the FRCP to function in a consultant and resource-facilitator role,
- clarify the lead coordinator role and responsibilities for executing a recovering servicemember's comprehensive plan,
- identify the business requirements for technical tools to support the interagency comprehensive plan, and
- accelerate existing information-sharing efforts for care coordination.

The Joint Executive Council provisionally approved the six recommendations, but withheld final approval pending receipt of additional information from the task force, such as an estimate of resources required to implement the recommendations, as well as details of the proposed interagency governance structure. The Joint Executive Council instructed the task force to present the additional information to them in another decision briefing, which was scheduled for September 20, 2012. Absent final approval from the Joint Executive Council, the task force's next step was to hold a status briefing for the DOD and VA Secretaries on September 10, 2012, to discuss the task force's recommended course of action for care coordination.

Given the inability of past task forces to effect changes that better align DOD and VA care coordination and case management policies, it is too soon to determine the full effect of the departments' efforts to manage care coordination services regarding outcomes for recovering servicemembers and veterans. Although VA and DOD appear to be moving in a positive direction on care coordination, notable barriers remain:

- There is concern as to whether the Joint Executive Council can effectively lead the effort to realign VA's and DOD's care coordination policy. Some high-ranking and cognizant DOD officials we talked with expressed concerns that the recently merged Joint Executive Council may not have the capability to effectively monitor the actions taken by DOD and VA to implement the task force's recommendations. Some officials we talked with viewed the council as taking too long to resolve issues due to both the infrequency of its meetings[64] and the difficulties DOD and VA members have in agreeing with one another.
- Following approval of its recommended course of action, task force documents indicate that a detailed plan will be completed by July 2013. VA's task force cochair stated that some aspects of the planned changes could take years to implement, particularly as they transition

existing enrollees of programs affected by significant revisions. For example, VA intends to conduct a case-by-case review of every FRCP enrollee before modifying the FRCP to function in a consultant and resource-facilitator role, according to VA's Task Force cochair.

- One of the most fundamental challenges to resolving care coordination problems is the issue of obtaining the cooperation of the military services to implement a new approach to care coordination and case management, especially in light of past difficulties of working in concert with DOD and VA programs and policies. DOD and VA leadership officials stated that even if new solutions and policies were to be approved by the departments, changes would be made only if the individual military services implement the new policies as directed by the Secretary of Defense. Several DOD and VA officials identified concurrence and support of the military services as the most difficult element to achieve. Ultimately, the military services' compliance with the departments' agreed-upon strategy for care coordination and case management programs will determine how seamlessly recovering servicemembers and veterans will be able to navigate the recovery care continuum.

CONCLUSION

The deficiencies exposed at Walter Reed in 2007 served as a catalyst compelling DOD and VA to address a host of problems that complicate the course of a wounded, ill, and injured servicemember's recovery, rehabilitation, and return to active duty or civilian life. We believe strongly and have reported already that fixing the long-standing and complex problems highlighted in the wake of the Walter Reed media accounts as expeditiously as possible is critical to ensuring high-quality care for returning servicemembers and veterans. We continue to believe that the departments' success ultimately depends on sustained attention, systematic oversight, and sufficient resources from both DOD and VA. However, this has not yet occurred, and as a result, after 5 years, recovering servicemembers and veterans are still facing problems as they navigate the recovery care continuum, including access to some of the programs designed to assist them. The transition period from DOD's to VA's health care system is particularly critical, as servicemembers continue to experience delays in the disability evaluation system and the departments continue to use methods other than a common information technology system to share servicemembers' health information. Until these problems are resolved, recovering servicemembers and veterans may still face difficulties getting the services they need to maximize their potential when they return to active duty or transition to civilian life.

Initially, departmental leadership exhibited focus and commitment—through the Senior Oversight Committee—to addressing problems related to case management and care coordination, disability evaluation systems, and data sharing between DOD and VA. However, over time, waning leadership attention, a failure to oversee critical wounded warrior functions and programs, limited resources, and the inability to achieve a collaborative environment— particularly with care coordination—have impeded the departments' ability to fully resolve these problems.

A key element in resolving current care coordination issues in particular is eliciting the cooperation of the military services, which are responsible for implementing various wounded warrior programs and ensuring that these programs operate as intended—which has sometimes not been the case, as with the RCP. Also, absent clear direction and central oversight and accountability among the military services' wounded warrior programs, true cooperation and program effectiveness may be in jeopardy.

We believe that at the heart of the problem is the need for strong and unwavering leadership to bring about changes that best serve our nation's recovering servicemembers and veterans.

This leadership should be united across both DOD and VA and centered on the individual servicemember's or veteran's recovery. Many task forces—including the VA/DOD Warrior Care and Coordination Task Force and the Recovering Warrior Task Force—have already attempted to bring a spirit of cooperativeness and clear direction and purpose among the different programs providing services to this population. However, to date, these efforts have not fully resolved key issues, and our nation's recovering servicemembers and veterans continue to face obstacles and challenges, especially as they transition from DOD's to VA's health care system.

Certainly, the fluidity and focus of the departments' leadership over the last several years, especially related to care coordination, have added to the challenges of developing consistent policy, effective oversight, and mechanisms to monitor progress and hold programs accountable. The departments have recently taken steps to improve problems related to care coordination, disability evaluations, and the electronic sharing of health records, through concerted efforts to coordinate on policy, increase staffing resources, and provide control over the budget, respectively.

However, it is too early to determine the effectiveness of these efforts, and sustained leadership attention will be critical to their success. The need to fully resolve remaining problems is urgent as there will be an increasing demand for services from both DOD and VA as the current conflicts come to an end. If not resolved now, these same problems will persist into the future for recovering servicemembers and veterans.

RECOMMENDATIONS FOR EXECUTIVE ACTION

To ensure that servicemembers have equitable access to the military services' wounded warrior programs, including the RCP, and to establish central accountability for these programs, we recommend that the Secretary of Defense establish or designate an office to centrally oversee and monitor the activities of the military services' wounded warrior programs to include the following:

- Develop consistent eligibility criteria to ensure that similarly situated recovering servicemembers from different military services have uniform access to these programs.
- Direct the military services' wounded warrior programs to fully comply with the policies governing care coordination and case management programs and any future changes to these policies.
- Develop a common mechanism to systematically monitor the performance of the wounded warrior programs—to include the establishment of common terms and definitions—and report this information on a biannual basis to the Armed Services Committees of the House of Representatives and the Senate.

To ensure that persistent challenges with care coordination, disability evaluation, and the electronic sharing of health records are fully resolved, we recommend that the Secretaries of Defense and Veterans Affairs ensure that these issues receive sustained leadership attention and collaboration at the highest levels with a singular focus on what is best for the individual servicemember or veteran to ensure continuity of care and a seamless transition from DOD to VA.

This should include holding the Joint Executive Council accountable for

- ensuring that key issues affecting recovering servicemembers and veterans get sufficient consideration, including recommendations made by the Warrior Care and Coordination Task Force and the Recovering Warrior Task Force;
- developing mechanisms for making joint policy decisions;
- involving the appropriate decision-makers for timely implementation of policy; and
- establishing mechanisms to systematically oversee joint initiatives and ensure that outcomes and goals are identified and achieved.

AGENCY COMMENTS AND OUR EVALUATION

DOD and VA reviewed a draft of this report and provided comments. DOD and VA also provided technical comments, which we incorporated as appropriate.

DOD concurred with specific components of our first recommendation regarding the establishment of central accountability for the military services' wounded warrior programs. In particular, DOD agreed that a single office should have oversight responsibility for the military services' wounded warrior programs and that these programs should fully comply with the policies governing care coordination and case management programs and any future changes to these policies.

However, DOD only partially concurred with other components of our first recommendation—that DOD develop consistent eligibility criteria for enrollment in wounded warrior programs and that DOD establish a common mechanism to systematically monitor the performance of these programs. In its comments, DOD explained that the three military service Secretaries should have the ability to control entrance criteria into their wounded warrior programs and added that it does not believe that differences in eligibility criteria for these programs results in noticeable differences in access to these programs by recovering servicemembers or their families. DOD did not offer a rationale, however, as to why the military service Secretaries should unilaterally determine eligibility criteria for their wounded warrior programs, other than to suggest that flexibility is important and necessary. Moreover, as we have reported, DOD does not systematically assess or monitor these programs across the department, and as a result, we believe that DOD has no basis to assert that there are no noticeable differences in access to these programs. Overall, we believe that similarly situated wounded, ill, and injured servicemembers should be given the same access to wounded warrior programs and the assistance these programs provide, regardless of their branch of military service.

With respect to developing a common mechanism to systematically monitor the performance of the wounded warrior programs, DOD responded that the Interagency Care and Coordination Committee will conduct an inventory of all wounded warrior programs to identify duplication and areas for gaining efficiencies. In commenting on our recommendation to also report its performance information on the wounded warrior programs to the Armed Services Committees on a biannual basis, DOD stated that the department reports progress through the Joint Executive Council's annual strategic planning report and any additional reporting would be redundant and of limited value. We disagree. The Joint Executive Council's strategic planning and annual reports focus on joint efforts between the departments and do not report on the performance of the military services' wounded warrior programs. Therefore, we do not believe that the performance information on the wounded warrior programs would be redundant or of limited value given that the department itself is currently unable to systematically determine how well these programs are functioning. As we reported, one of the key problems hindering a department-wide assessment of these programs is the lack of common terms and definitions used by the military services. Although DOD acknowledges that this is an issue, it asserts that it has instituted some common definitions through the Senior Oversight Committee and through its instruction for the RCP and that it will work towards a common understanding and use of these approved definitions. Although we are aware of efforts to define some terms, on the basis of our work, it does not appear that the military services are using them consistently. Therefore, substantial progress towards a common understanding and use will be critical to the department's ability to oversee these programs.

DOD did not respond directly to our recommendation for developing a common mechanism for performance measurement, which we found is not systematically conducted across the wounded warrior programs. During our collection of performance data from the wounded warrior programs, we found that the programs vary in their ability to report performance outcome measures on the basis of what each program chooses to track. In addition, we found that some of the programs had difficulty reporting basic data, such as enrollment numbers, and only compiled these data following our request—sometimes taking about 5 months to do so. Lastly, our recommendation is consistent with the call of the Interagency Care and Coordination Committee that the military programs develop more useful quantitative and qualitative metrics that would effectively demonstrate their performance. Until DOD takes the necessary steps to assess these programs department-wide, it will never know with certitude whether these programs are meeting the needs of its recovering servicemember population.

DOD and VA both concurred with our second recommendation that the departments ensure that care coordination, disability evaluation, and electronic health record sharing receive sustained leadership attention and collaboration at the highest levels, with a singular focus on what is best for the individual servicemember or veteran to ensure continuity of care and a seamless transition from DOD to VA.

In addition to its comments on our recommendation, VA asserted that the care coordination challenges facing both departments are broader and more complex than issues concerning just the FRCP and RCP and that our overall analysis and conclusions are over simplified. VA stated that through its recently formed task force, both departments identified over 40 programs that provide some level of coordination or management of care and services across the continuum of care and acknowledged that there is no common operational picture that facilitates collaborative planning or situational awareness. We agree that the care coordination challenges are broader and more complex than the FRCP and RCP. Specifically, in October 2011, we recommended that the departments strengthen functional integration across all care coordination and case management programs to reduce redundancy and overlap.[65] Similarly, our current recommendation is broad and does not focus exclusively on these two programs as our review also included other programs, such as the military services' wounded warrior programs, VA's Liaison for Healthcare Program, and VA's OEF/OIF/OND Care Management Program. The scope of our review was directed by Congress, who required us to report on the progress DOD and VA in implementing the programs involved with the care, management, and transition of wounded, ill, and injured servicemembers that they established. Our specific discussion of the FRCP and RCP served to illustrate, until recently, a continued lack of collaboration between the departments to better align these programs and better serve recovering servicemembers and veterans. Furthermore, during detailed discussions with top-level VA and DOD officials, they focused on the FRCP and RCP issue as the main sticking point in achieving coordination and cooperation among the two departments with respect to care coordination and case management. We are encouraged that the departments are now taking steps to identify all programs that need better alignment and integration. However, as we have stated, the key to resolving this and other problems is the need for strong and unwavering leadership that is united across both departments and focused on the individual servicemember's or veteran's recovery.

VA also suggested further clarifications to our report.

- VA suggested that we clarify that while the VA Liaison for Healthcare Program facilitates the transfer of recovering servicemembers from DOD's to VA's health care system, it is a DOD or VA treatment team that determines if the servicemember is medically ready to begin the transition process. VA also suggested that we add that that the OEF/OIF/OND Care Management Program screens all returning combat veterans for case management services. We incorporated VA's suggested changes.
- VA disagrees with a DOD-attributed statement that the Joint Executive Council historically has not driven policy decision making and that, at times, decisions were taken directly to the DOD and VA Secretaries for resolution. The statement that we attribute to the DOD official relates to the period prior to the integration of the Senior Oversight Committee with the Joint Executive Council. As mentioned in the report, it is too early to ascertain whether the newly merged Joint Executive Council will be able to make decisions and drive policy changes in DOD and VA.
- VA provided clarification about how the Joint Executive Council is currently providing oversight and accountability for wounded warrior issues that were once addressed by the Senior Oversight Committee. We recognize the effort that the Joint Executive Council is now making to track wounded warrior issues, including the integrated disability evaluation system and care coordination. However, we have not had the opportunity to review this tracking mechanism now in place to comment on its effectiveness.
- VA asserts that the size of the overlap between the FRCP and RCP population is fairly small. Although the number of seriously injured servicemembers may be comparatively small, this situation has been and continues to be a major concern in that these individuals and their families represent a highly vulnerable population. Further, during our review, one high-level DOD official we spoke with characterized the

FRCP/RCP overlap as the most difficult policy issue to resolve. While we understand that DOD and VA now intend to harmonize care coordination policies within a broader context of interdepartmental care coordination and case management practice, many of the proposed revisions—including the role to be played by the FRCP—are neither fully developed nor implemented by the separate DOD and VA programs at this time.

- In our report, we explain that VA declined DOD's requests to discuss care coordination and case management policy issues—for the better part of 1 year—on the basis that VA was conducting an internal review of its care coordination and case management activities. In its comments, VA stated that the use of the word "decline" is misleading, and suggested that we change our text to state that VA asked DOD to defer collaboration until the internal review was conducted. Despite VA's characterization that our statement is misleading, we maintain that this finding was based on remarks made by high-level DOD officials that were subsequently corroborated by senior VA officials.

Randall B. Williamson
Director, Health Care

APPENDIX I: ENROLLMENT AND POPULATIONS FOR SELECT DEPARTMENT OF DEFENSE AND DEPARTMENT OF VETERANS AFFAIRS PROGRAMS

Both the Department of Defense (DOD) and the Department of Veterans Affairs (VA) operate care coordination[1] and case management[2] programs designed to assist servicemembers and veterans as they navigate the recovery care continuum, from acute medical treatment and stabilization, through rehabilitation, to reintegration—either back to active duty or to the civilian community as a veteran.

This appendix describes selected DOD and VA programs and includes data on enrollment and population characteristics as well as the type of information each program tracks on referrals.

DOD WOUNDED WARRIOR PROGRAMS

Within DOD, each military service has established its own wounded warrior program or a complement of programs[3] to assist wounded, ill, and injured servicemembers during their recovery and rehabilitation, and to help with the transition back to active duty or to civilian life.[4] Wounded warrior programs range in size from the largest, the Army's Warrior Transition Units and Community-Based Warrior Transition Units, with 18,762 enrollees served in fiscal year 2011, to the smallest, the Navy Safe Harbor Program, with 784 enrollees served in fiscal year 2011. (See table 4 for a list of the DOD wounded warrior programs and enrollment for fiscal year 2011.)

Programs differ in their organization and function. For example, two of the wounded warrior programs—the Army's Warrior Transition Units and the Marine Corps Wounded Warrior Regiment—are organized under separate military commands, which means that wounded, ill, and injured servicemembers enrolled in these programs may be removed from their parent units or commands and assigned or attached to a separate unit or regiment that provides command and control[5] over the recovering servicemember as well as administrative support. These servicemembers may be housed in separate barracks while receiving medical care and waiting to transition back to active duty or civilian life. The other wounded warrior programs do not assign or attach servicemembers to a separate command structure, but provide services while recovering servicemembers remain with their parent units. The services provided by the wounded warrior programs also vary. A servicemember may receive either case management or care coordination services or both, depending on how the military service's wounded warrior program is structured.

For example, the Navy Safe Harbor Program only provides care coordination services and does not have a case management component, whereas the Marine Corps Wounded Warrior Regiment provides all servicemembers with both case management and care coordination services. A further distinction is whether or not a program serves veterans as well as servicemembers. For example, the Army Warrior Transition Units do not serve veterans, but eligible veterans are served through the Army Wounded Warrior Program.

The remainder of the wounded warrior programs continue to provide support to any enrollee who needs services even after the enrollee has transitioned to veteran status.

Table 4. Military Services' Wounded Warrior Programs: Enrollment for Fiscal Year 2011

Military services' wounded warrior program	Number enrolled, as of fiscal year 2011
Army	
Army Warrior Care and Transition Program: Warrior Transition Units and Community-Based Warrior Transition Units[a,b]	18,762
Army Warrior Care and Transition Program: Army Wounded Warrior Program[b]	9,738
Navy/Coast Guard	
Navy Safe Harbor Program[c]	784
Air Force	
Air Force Wounded Warrior Program[d]	1,386
Air Force Recovery Care Program	1,804
Marine Corps	
Marine Corps Wounded Warrior Regiment[e,f]	2,155
United States Special Operations Command[g]	
United States Special Operations Command's Care Coalition	4,570

Source: GAO analysis of military services' wounded warrior program information.

[a] Enrollment data include servicemembers who were in the Army Warrior Care and Transition Program at any point during the fiscal year, not the population on a specific date.

[b] Enrollees may include servicemembers who are dually enrolled in the Army Warrior Care and Transition Program and Army Wounded Warrior Program.

[c] Enrollment numbers represent all enrollees being served by the program as of December 31, rather than as of the end of each fiscal year.

[d] Servicemembers may be dually enrolled in the Air Force Wounded Warrior Program and the Air Force Recovery Care Program. The enrollment data presented here only reflect servicemembers who are enrolled in the Air Force Wounded Warrior Program.

[e] According to a Wounded Warrior Regiment official, the Wounded Warrior Regiment does not have "enrollees," rather the program assigns and attaches Marines to the program.

[f] Total enrollment does not include Wounded Warrior Regiment enrollees who are not assigned or attached to a Wounded Warrior Regiment site. Many wounded, ill, and injured Marines are supported by the Wounded Warrior Regiment while remaining with their parent unit.

[g] Enrollees of the United States Special Operations Command's Care Coalition Recovery Program may also be enrolled in a military service's wounded warrior program on the basis of their branch of service, but the United States Special Operations Command's Care Coalition Recovery Program takes the lead for providing nonclinical case management.

Army Warrior Care and Transition Program

The Army's Warrior Care and Transition Program, which was established in May 2007,[6] consists of two components that support the recovery process for wounded, ill, and injured servicemembers—the Warrior Transition Units[7] and the Army Wounded Warrior Program.

The Army operates a number of warrior transition units located at Army installations across the country. Recovering servicemembers who are attached or assigned to a warrior transition unit generally are housed in barracks and receive medical care, rehabilitative services, professional development and clinical and nonclinical case management services in order to help them in their transition back to active duty or to the civilian community.

Army Warrior Transition Units vary in size and functionality, including community-based warrior transition units,[8] which primarily serve Reserve Component servicemembers.[9] In fiscal year 2011, there were a total of 14,906 recovering servicemembers assigned or attached to 29 warrior transition units and 3,856 recovering servicemembers assigned or attached to 10 community-based warrior transition units. (See table 5.)

According to Army policy, recovering servicemembers assigned or attached to the units are expected to require 6 months or more of rehabilitative care or require complex medical management.

The Army Wounded Warrior Program [10] was established in April 2004 to assist severely wounded, ill, and injured servicemembers, their families, and caregivers. Army Wounded Warrior Program enrollees are assigned an Advocate who provides nonclinical care coordination services, which include assisting enrollees with benefit information, career guidance, finances, and the integrated disability evaluation system (IDES) process. Recovering servicemembers are eligible for Army Wounded Warrior Program services if they have, or are expected to receive, an Army disability rating of 30 percent or greater in one or more specific categories or a combined rating of 50 percent or greater for conditions that are the result of combat or are combat-related.

The most severely wounded, ill, or injured servicemembers who are assigned to warrior transition units are also enrolled in the Army Wounded Warrior Program. The Army Wounded Warrior Program also provides services to veterans. In fiscal year 2011, nearly three-fourths of the population (6,953) were veterans. (See table 6.)

Table 5. Army Warrior Care and Transition Program Enrollment Populations and Characteristics, Fiscal Years 2008 through 2011

	Fiscal year			
	2008	*2009*	*2010*	*2011*
Program enrollment for Warrior Transition Units and Community-Based Warrior Transition Units				
Total enrollment[a,b]	*20,878*	*19,238*	*18,647*	*18,762*
Active Duty	13,558	11,771	9,560	9,160
National Guard[c]	4,761	4,839	5,860	5,857
Reservists[c]	2,559	2,628	3,227	3,745
Population characteristics				
Enrollees with combat-related conditions[d]	2,523	2,033	1,788	1,984
Enrollees with non-combat-related conditions[e]	18,355	17,205	16,859	16,778
Enrollees who left the program				
Returned to active duty[f]	4,366	4,279	4,664	5,349
Transitioned to veteran status[g]	5,125	5,938	4,027	3,448
Left for other reasons[h]	146	200	159	148
Referrals				
Total number of servicemembers referred to the program[i]	*20,878*	*19,238*	*18,647*	*18,762*
Warrior Transition Unit enrollment				
Total enrollment in Warrior Transition Units[a,b]	*18,038*	*16,203*	*14,921*	*14,906*
Active Duty	13,511	11,686	9,456	9,058
National Guard[c]	2,864	2,807	3,336	3,354
Reservists[c]	1,663	1,710	2,129	2,494
Population characteristics				
Enrollees with combat-related conditions[d]	2,231	1,798	1,569	1,760
Enrollees with non-combat-related conditions[e]	15,807	14,405	13,352	13,146
Enrollees who left the program				
Returned to active duty[f]	3,613	3,653	3,803	4,259
Transitioned to veteran status[g]	4,706	5,445	3,700	3,167
Left for other reasons[h]	139	184	146	135
Community-Based Warrior Transition Unit enrollment				
Total enrollment in Community-Based Warrior Transition Units[a,b,j]	*2,840*	*3,035*	*3,726*	*3,856*
Active Duty	47	85	104	102
National Guard[c]	1,897	2,032	2,524	2,503
Reservists[c]	896	918	1,098	1,251
Population characteristics				
Enrollees with combat-related conditionsd	292	235	219	224
Enrollees with non-combat-related conditionse	2,548	2,800	3,507	3,632
Enrollees who left the program				
Returned to active dutyf	753	626	861	1,090

Table 5. (Continued)

	Fiscal year			
	2008	*2009*	*2010*	*2011*
Transitioned to veteran statusg	419	493	327	281
Left for other reasonsh	7	16	13	13

Source: GAO analysis of Army Warrior Care and Transition Program data.

Notes: The Army Warrior Care and Transition Program's Warrior Transition Units and Community-Based Warrior Transition Units serve Active, Guard, and Reserve Component servicemembers. The program does not serve veterans.

[a] Enrollment data include servicemembers who were in the Army Warrior Care and Transition Program at any point during the fiscal year, not the population on a specific date.

[b] Enrollees may include servicemembers who are dually enrolled in the Army Warrior Care and Transition Program and the Army Wounded Warrior Program.

[c] National Guard and Reservists enrolled in the Army Warrior Care and Transition Program must be on active-duty orders in order to participate in the program.

[d] Enrollees with combat-related conditions only include those enrollees medically evacuated from a combat zone with identified battle injuries. Other combat-related conditions, such as posttraumatic stress disorder, may not have required medical evacuation from a combat zone and therefore would not be captured in the data provided. In addition, prior battle injuries not related to the servicemember's current medical diagnosis would also be excluded from the data. Battle injury is defined as damage or harm sustained by personnel during or as a result of battle conditions.

[e] Enrollees with non-combat-related conditions include all enrollees who were not medically evacuated from a combat zone and those who are identified as having nonbattle injuries.

[f] Enrollees who exit the program by returning to duty also include Guard or Reserve Components who are released from active duty, but not medically separated from military service.

[g] Enrollees who transition to veteran status include only enrollees who are medically separated from military service.

[h] Enrollees are considered to have left the Army Warrior Care and Transition Program's Warrior Transition Units for "other" reasons, including death or as a result of military legal actions. This category also includes those enrollees with incomplete information about why they left the program.

[i] According to Army Warrior Care and Transition Program officials, the program only tracks referral information for program enrollees. Therefore, the program does not have data on servicemembers who were referred, but never enrolled into the program.

[j] The Army's Community-Based Warrior Transition Units are populated only by servicemembers who transfer to the Community-Based Units from their original assignment to a Warrior Transition Unit. According to Army Warrior Care and Transition Program officials, the first 60 days of recovery are typically spent in a Warrior Transition Unit. After the initial recovery period, a decision is made about whether the servicemember should be transferred to a community-based unit. Data provided in the table reflect the most recent location recorded for each enrollee.

Table 6. Army Wounded Warrior Program Enrollment Populations and Characteristics, Fiscal Years 2008 through 2011

	Fiscal year			
	2008	2009	2010	2011
Program enrollment for Army Wounded Warrior Program				
Total enrollment [a,b]	3,813	6,473	8,454	9,738
Servicemembers	2,037	3,377	3,354	2,785
Active Duty	1,249	2,252	1,954	1,210
National Guardc	562	794	985	1,091
Reservists[c]	226	331	415	484
Veterans	1,776	3,096	5,100	6,953
Population characteristics				
Enrollees with combat-related conditions	3,233	5,503	7,082	8,001
Enrollees with non-combat-related conditions	544	875	1,104	1,184
Enrollees with conditions not classified as either combat- or non-combat-related[d]	36	95	268	553
Enrollees who changed duty status or left the program				
Returned to active duty[e]	117	80	59	47
Transitioned to veteran status[f]	958	1,574	1,539	1,100
Left for other reasons[g]	10	24	21	3
Referrals and assists				
Total number of servicemembers referred to the program	3,106	4,199	3,993	3,364
Servicemembers referred and enrolled in the program	2,037	3,377	3,354	2,785
Servicemembers referred and assisted, but not enrolled in the program[h]	969	822	639	579
Total number of veterans referred to the program	2,568	3,617	5,554	7,291
Veterans referred and enrolled in the program	1,776	3,096	5,100	6,953
Veterans referred and assisted, but not enrolled in the program	792	521	454	338

Source: GAO analysis of Army Wounded Warrior Program data.

[a] Enrollment data include servicemembers and veterans who were served by the program at any point during the fiscal year, not the population being served on a specific date.

[b] Enrollees also may be enrolled in the Army's Warrior Transition Units or Community-Based Warrior Transition Units.

[c] Enrollment is counted in this category only for National Guard and Reservists who were on active duty orders during the designated fiscal year. According to Army Wounded Warrior Program officials, National Guard and Reservists who were demobilized previous to the designated fiscal year are considered veterans.

[d] Enrollees considered to have "conditions not classified as either combat- or non-combat-related" include enrollees who have yet to complete the physical disability

evaluation process and therefore do not have verification of whether or not their conditions are combat-related.

[e] Army Wounded Warrior Program officials said that the program does not specifically track whether or when an enrollee returns to active duty. However, data on duty status are available for those enrollees who are also enrolled in the Army's Warrior Transition Units or Community-Based Warrior Transition Unit, as provided in the table.

[f] Army Wounded Warrior Program officials said that the program does not specifically track whether or when an enrollee transitions to veteran status because it has no impact on enrollees' eligibility for the program and whether they leave the program. Rather, these data have been derived by the program by counting the number of enrolled servicemembers who received a certificate of release or discharge from active duty within each fiscal year.

[g] Enrollees considered to have "left for other reasons" include those who died while enrolled in the Army Wounded Warrior Program.

[h] The data include those enrollees who were later found ineligible for the program and were disenrolled, but assisted during their initial period of enrollment. These ineligible enrollees were not included in the program's count of total enrollees. Additionally, some servicemembers who were referred to the Wounded Warrior Program and provided short-term, informal assistance are not included in the data because they are not tracked by the program.

Navy Safe Harbor Program

The Navy Safe Harbor Program office was established in 2005. Over time, this office expanded its reach and mission, and in 2008 the program became responsible for nonclinical care coordination and oversight of all severely (and high-risk nonseverely) wounded, ill, and injured Sailors and Coast Guardsmen.[11]

Recovering servicemembers enrolled in the program are assigned to nonmedical care managers who are geographically dispersed at major military treatment facilities and Veterans Affairs polytrauma medical centers.

The program's nonmedical care managers assist enrollees with services such as pay and personnel, legal, housing, as well as education and training benefits. In addition, enrollees obtain support from centrally located experts in transition and benefits assistance, such as a liaison to the Department of Labor and a Navy Staff Judge Advocate. Recovering servicemembers enrolled in the program are enrolled for life and, if desired, receive support from Navy Safe Harbor personnel after they transition to veteran status. (See table 7.)

Table 7. Navy Safe Harbor Program Enrollment Populations and Characteristics, Fiscal Years 2008 through 2011

	Fiscal year			
	2008	2009	2010	2011
Program enrollment for Navy Safe Harbor Program				
Total enrollment[a]	255	434	576	784
Servicemembers	144	236	271	391
Active Duty	77	129	152	254
Reservists	67	107	119	137
Veterans	111	198	305	393
Population characteristics				
Enrollees with combat-related conditions	130	166	193	239
Enrollees with non-combat-related conditions	125	268	383	545
Enrollees who changed duty status or left the program				
Returned to active duty	ND	ND	ND	113
Transitioned to veteran status	ND	91[b]	338[b]	142
Left for other reasons	0	0	0	1
Referrals and assists				
Total number of servicemembers and veterans referred to the program[c]	304	296	370	475
Servicemembers and veterans referred and enrolled in the program	255	179	142	208
Servicemembers and veterans referred and assisted, but not enrolled in the program	74	417	330	199
Servicemembers and veterans referred but not enrolled in or assisted by the program	0	0	2	73

Legend: ND indicates that no data are available.

Source: GAO analysis of Navy Safe Harbor Program data.

[a] Enrollment numbers represent all enrollees being served by the program as of December 31, rather than as of the end of each fiscal year.

[b] According to a Navy Safe Harbor Program official, the database used to capture information about the duty status of enrollees did not have the ability to track dates when servicemembers transitioned to veteran status until the system was upgraded in 2010. At that point, the program moved all enrollees who had previously medically retired to a veteran status. Therefore, the number of enrollees who transitioned to veteran status in fiscal year 2010 includes both servicemembers who transitioned to veteran status within the fiscal year and servicemembers who transitioned to veteran status during the previous fiscal years.

[c] The database used to capture referral information for the Navy Safe Harbor Program does not distinguish servicemembers from veterans referred to the program. Rather, the referral information provided for servicemembers also includes any veterans who were referred to the program.

Table 8. Air Force Wounded Warrior Program Enrollment Populations and Characteristics, Fiscal Years 2008 through 2011

	Fiscal year			
	2008	2009	2010	*2011*
Program enrollment for Air Force Wounded Warrior Program				
Total enrollment[a]	194	451	836	*1,386*
Servicemembers	160	388	703	1,143
Active Duty	103	256	463	783
National Guard	32	60	123	194
Reservists	25	72	117	166
Veterans	34	63	133	243
Population characteristics				
Enrollees with combat-related conditions	187	442	804	1,327
Enrollees with non-combat-related conditions	7	9	32	59
Enrollees who changed duty status or left the program				
Returned to active duty	4	22	65	128
Transitioned to veteran status	157	329	532	786
Referrals and assists				
Total number of servicemembers referred to the program	146	357	724	*1,176*
Servicemembers referred and enrolled in the program	145	337	645	1,071
Servicemembers referred and assisted, but not enrolled in the program[b]	1	20	79	105
Servicemembers referred but not enrolled in or assisted by the program	0	0	0	0
Total number of veterans referred to the program	34	63	133	*243*
Veterans referred and enrolled in the program	34	63	133	243
Veterans referred and assisted, but not enrolled in the program	NA	NA	NA	NA
Veterans referred but not enrolled in or assisted by the program	0	0	0	0

Legend: NA indicates that the category is not applicable to the program.

Source: GAO analysis of Air Force Wounded Warrior Program data.

[a] Servicemembers may be dually enrolled in the Air Force Recovery Care Program and the Air Force Wounded Warrior Program. The enrollment data presented here only reflect servicemembers who are enrolled in the Air Force Wounded Warrior Program.

[b] According to Air Force Wounded Warrior Program officials, because the program only serves servicemembers with combat-related conditions, most referrals come from casualty reports and the disability evaluation process, where it is determined whether a servicemember's wound, illness, and injury are combat-related. Once the determination is made, servicemembers are enrolled into the program.

Air Force Warrior and Survivor Care Program

The Air Force Warrior and Survivor Care Program supports wounded, ill, and injured servicemembers through its Air Force Wounded Warrior Program and the Air Force Recovery Care Program.[12] The Air Force Wounded Warrior Program was established in June 2005 to provide nonclinical case management to Airmen, Air National Guard, and Reserve Component servicemembers who have combat-related illnesses or injuries. Each enrolled servicemember is assigned a nonmedical care manager, who serves as an advocate for enrollees to obtain services from agencies and organizations that support the needs of enrolled servicemembers, their families and caregivers. The Air Force Wounded Warrior Program continues to provide services to enrollees once they transition to veteran status. (See table 8.)

The Air Force Recovery Care Program was established in November 2008 to provide nonclinical care coordination services for seriously ill and injured Airmen, Air National Guard, and Reserve Component servicemembers. Each enrolled servicemember is assigned a care coordinator who oversees the coordination of services and assists enrollees' with nonclinical needs, such as employment and benefits. These care coordinators also work with enrolled servicemembers to develop their recovery plans and career goals. Enrollees who have combat-related illness or injuries are concurrently enrolled in the Air Force Wounded Warrior Program. For example, in fiscal year 2011, almost 300 Air Force Recovery Care Program enrollees were also either tracked or actively assisted by the Air Force Wounded Warrior Program. (See table 9.)

Marine Corps Wounded Warrior Regiment

The Marine Corps established the Wounded Warrior Regiment in May 2007 to provide and facilitate assistance to wounded, ill, and injured Marines and their family members throughout the recovery process. The Wounded Warrior Regiment is a single command that oversees nonmedical care for the total Marine force, including Active Duty, Reserve, retired, and veteran Marines. The regiment enrolls Marines regardless of whether they have combat- or non-combat-related conditions. The regiment commands the operation of two wounded warrior battalions and 14 detachments located at 12 principal military treatment facilities and four Veterans Affairs polytrauma medical centers across the United States and overseas.

Table 9. Air Force Recovery Care Program Enrollment Populations and Characteristics, Fiscal Years 2008 through 2011

	Fiscal year			
	2008	2009	2010	2011
Program enrollment for Air Force Recovery Care Program				
Total enrollment [a]	*ND*	*ND*	*ND*	1,804
Servicemembers	ND	ND	ND	ND
National Guard	ND	ND	ND	ND
Reservists	ND	ND	ND	ND
Veterans	ND	ND	ND	ND
Others[b]	ND	ND	ND	251
Population characteristics				
Enrollees with combat-related conditions	ND	ND	ND	316
Enrollees with non-combat-related conditions	ND	ND	ND	782
Enrollees who changed duty status or left the program				
Returned to active duty	ND	ND	ND	288
Transitioned to veteran status	ND	ND	ND	394
Left for other reasons	ND	ND	ND	ND
Referrals and assists				
Total number of servicemembers referred to the program	*ND*	*ND*	*ND*	1,804

Legend: ND indicates that no data are available.

Source: GAO analysis of Air Force Recovery Care Program data.

Notes: According to Air Force Recovery Care Program officials, the program did not routinely track certain data about the program, because these data were not required to be collected by the DOD policy that governs the program. In addition, the original Air Force Recovery Care program requirements did not include provisions for data collection. The officials told us that a data-collection tool is being developed and that requirements for data collection would be finalized by the beginning of July 2012. The officials anticipate the new tool will be operational by January 2013.

[a] Enrollees may also be enrolled in the Air Force's Wounded Warrior Program.

[b] The Air Force Recovery Care Program serves some servicemembers from other military services.

A Marine enrolled in the regiment can either stay with his or her parent unit and be supported by the regiment, or be assigned or attached to one of the regiment's battalions and detachments, depending on their specific needs. Generally, Marines who require more than 90 days of medical treatment or rehabilitation are assigned or attached to a battalion or detachment. The District Injured Support Cells Program is the component of the Wounded Warrior Regiment that provides services to veterans.13 District Injured Support Coordinators are located at 30 sites across the United States to provide support, including nonmedical care management to its enrollees. In fiscal year 2011, the District Injured Support Coordinators provided support to 1,488 veterans. (See table 10.)

Table 10. Marine Corps Wounded Warrior Regiment Enrollment Populations and Characteristics, Fiscal Years 2008 through 2011

	Fiscal year			
	2008	2009	2010	2011
Program enrollment for Marine Corps Wounded Warrior Regiment				
Total enrollmenta,b	810	725	634	2,155
Servicemembers	810	725	634	667
Active Duty	712	633	494	517
Reservists	98	92	140	150
Veterans served through District Injured Support Coordinatorsc	ND	ND	ND	1,488
Population characteristics				
Enrollees with combat-related conditionsd	216	105	115	224
Enrollees with non-combat-related conditionse	594	620	519	443
Enrollees who changed duty status or left the program				
Returned to active duty	35	38	84	94
Transitioned to veteran status	149	266	311	366
Left for other reasonse	ND	ND	ND	ND
Referrals				
Total number of servicemembers referred to the programf	ND	ND	ND	ND
Total number of veterans referred to District Injured Support Coordinatorsg	ND	ND	ND	ND

Legend: ND indicates that no data are available.

Source: GAO analysis of Marine Corps Wounded Warrior Regiment data.

[a] According to a Wounded Warrior Regiment official, the Wounded Warrior Regiment does not have "enrollees," rather the program assigns and attaches Marines to the program.

[b] Total enrollment does not include Wounded Warrior Regiment enrollees who are not assigned or attached to a Wounded Warrior Regiment site. Many wounded, ill, and injured Marines are supported by the Wounded Warrior Regiment while remaining with their parent unit.

[c] The District Injured Support Coordinators provide outreach and services to Reserve and veteran Marines located across the country.

[d] The data in this category do not include Marines attached to the Wounded Warrior Regiment who may have been wounded, fallen ill, or injured in a combat zone, but who were not medically evacuated from a combat zone.

[e] Although the Wounded Warrior Regiment was not able to provide data on the number of enrollees who left the Wounded Warrior Regiment for reasons other than returning to duty or transitioning to veteran status, according to a Wounded Warrior Regiment official, Marines attached to the Wounded Warrior Regiment have left the program for other reasons such as death or as a result of military legal actions taken against the Marine.

[f] According to a Marine Corps Wounded Warrior Regiment official, although a policy exists requiring referral information to be collected, the policy was not always enforced. According to this official, as of fiscal year 2012, the data are routinely collected.

[g] According to a Marine Corps Wounded Warrior Regiment official, the District Injured Support Coordinators initially served veterans on an ad hoc basis, so referral information was not collected.

Table 11. United States Special Operations Command's Care Coalition Enrollment Populations and Characteristics, Fiscal Years 2008 through 2011

	Fiscal year			
	2008	2009	2010	2011
Program enrollment for United States Special Operations Command's Care Coalition				
Total enrollment[a]	2,277[b]	2,532[b]	3,447	4,570
Servicemembers	1,594	1,741	2,475	3,518
National Guard	113	127	154	228
Reservists	193	196	206	232
Veterans	654	722	838	893
Others[c]	152	192	262	287
Population characteristics				
Enrollees with combat-related conditions[d]	1,693	1,803	2,415	2,879

	Fiscal year			
	2008	2009	2010	2011
Enrollees with non-combat-related conditions[d]	736	839	1,256	1,859
Enrollees who changed duty status				
Returned to active duty[e]	31	32	38	46
Transitioned to veteran status[e]	4	23	24	48
Referrals				
Total number of servicemembers referred to the program[f]	ND	ND	ND	ND
Total number of veterans referred to the program[f]	ND	ND	ND	ND

Legend: ND indicates that no data are available.

Source: GAO analysis of United States Special Operations Command's Care Coalition data.

[a] Enrollees of the United States Special Operations Command's Care Coalition Recovery Program may also be enrolled in a military service's wounded warrior program on the basis of their branch of service, but the United States Special Operations Command's Care Coalition Recovery Program takes the lead for providing nonclinical case management.

[b] According to a United States Special Operations Command's Care Coalition official, because of a change in the data system used to track enrollment, enrollment numbers provided for fiscal year 2008 include enrollees served by the program between October 1, 2007, and May 28, 2009. Enrollment numbers provided for fiscal year 2009 include an additional 255 servicemembers and veterans who enrolled in the program between May 28, 2009, and September 30, 2009.

[c] Others enrolled include civilians, surviving family members, and records with unknown information. According to a United States Special Operations Command's Care Coalition official, the program continues to provide and track services to surviving family members after an enrolled servicemember or veteran has died.

[d] According to a United States Special Operations Command's Care Coalition official, data provided on enrollees with either combat- or non-combat-related conditions also include some servicemembers who were either killed in action or died while enrolled in the program, and therefore were excluded from the total enrollment data. In addition, officials stated that the exact count for non-combat-related conditions may not be accurate, due to inaccuracies in record keeping.

[e] According to a United States Special Operations Command's Care Coalition official, the program did not begin tracking enrollee transition status and transition dates in an accessible format until January 2012. Therefore, information about the duty status and transition status is being updated by hand as an individual record is reviewed by program personnel, and the information provided may not be accurate.

[f] According to a United States Special Operations Command's Care Coalition official, the program has several methods of receiving referrals, but its primary source of referrals comes from casualty reports. The program does not track referral information because the Care Coalition does not have a field in its database to track this information. However, this official said that the Care Coalition could access this information by contacting the military services.

United States Special Operations Command's Care Coalition

The United States Special Operations Command established the Care Coalition in August 2005 to track, support, and advocate for Special Operations Force's wounded, ill, and injured servicemembers regardless of their duty status or whether their conditions are combat-related. (See table 11.) All enrollees are assigned an Advocate and are entitled to advocate services for life. Advocates assist enrollees with health care and financial benefits, transition processes, and link enrollees with needed government and nongovernment resources. Because the United States Special Operations Command's Care Coalition serves servicemembers from across the military services, it serves as a liaison with, and complements, the military services' wounded warrior programs.

United States Special Operations Command's Care Coalition enrollees are often concurrently enrolled in their own military service's wounded warrior program. However, according to a Care Coalition official, the Care Coalition serves as the lead program for case management and care coordination for dually enrolled servicemembers.

VA Case Management and Care Coordination Programs

VA operates a number of case management and care coordination programs that provide assistance to recovering servicemembers and veterans, including the Operation Enduring Freedom/Operation Iraqi Freedom/Operation New Dawn (OEF/OIF/OND) Care Management Program and the Federal Recovery Coordination Program (FRCP).[14] These two programs assist wounded servicemembers and veterans to navigate the recovery care continuum.

OEF/OIF/OND Care Management Program

The OEF/OIF/OND Care Management Program was established in March 2007 to provide case management to wounded, ill, and injured servicemembers and veterans who screen positive for the need for case management or request case management services. (See table 12). Each of

VA's 152 Medical Centers (VAMC) has an OEF/OIF/OND Care Management team in place to manage patient care activities and ensure that servicemembers and veterans are receiving patient-centered, integrated care and benefits. Members of the OEF/OIF/OND Care Management team include: a Program Manager, Clinical Case Managers, and a Transition Patient Advocate.

Table 12. Operation Enduring Freedom/Operation Iraqi Freedom/ Operation New Dawn (OEF/OIF/OND) Care Management Program Enrollment Populations and Characteristics, Fiscal Years 2008 through 2011

	Fiscal year			
	2008[a]	2009[a]	2010	2011
Total enrollment[b]	2,463	7,048	49,145	50,255
Servicemembers[c]	152	590	2,069	2,505
Veterans	1,136	4,212	31,831	29,848
Others[d]	1,175	2,246	15,245	17,902
Population characteristics				
Enrollees with combat-related conditions[e]	1,214	2, 470	7,165	6,898
Enrollees with non-combat-related conditions[f]	212	676	3,115	3,188
Enrollees with conditions not classified as either combat- or non-combat-related[g]	200	880	4,820	4,072
Referrals				
Total number of servicemembers and veterans referred to the program by military treatment facilitiesh	2,130	4,474	7,172	6,686

Source: GAO analysis of OEF/OIF/OND Care Management Program data.

[a] According to OEF/OIF/OND Care Management Program officials, 2008 and 2009 data only include severely wounded, ill, and injured because the database only tracked this subpopulation of the program, which was the initial focus of the program's efforts. This population included, for example, those with severe burns, amputations, spinal cord injuries, or blindness, or more than one of these. Soon after the program was initiated, the Department of Veterans Affairs found that people returning from the conflicts in Iraq and Afghanistan required additional support, regardless of the severity of their injuries or illnesses. Therefore, policy was changed and the OEF/OIF/OND Care Management Program began tracking data on all those receiving case management services through their program.

[b] Total enrollment includes those who serve or served in National Guard and Reserve Components.

[c] The OEF/OIF/OND Care Management Program primarily serves veterans. Some servicemembers who are receiving treatment through a VA facility may also be enrolled in the program.

[d] Others include enrollees with unknown military status.

[e] Includes enrollees with battle injuries. According to OEF/OIF/OND Care Management Program officials, battle injuries are injuries sustained while in combat, such as a wound from an improvised explosive device.

[f] Includes enrollees with nonbattle injuries. According to OEF/OIF/OND Care Management Program officials, nonbattle injuries can include injuries sustained in a combat zone that are not directly related to combat.

[g] Includes enrollees with illnesses that may be classified as either combat-related or non-combatrelated. According to OEF/OIF/OND Care Management Program officials, the program tracks whether an enrollee's condition is a battle injury or a nonbattle injury, but not whether an illness is related to combat.

[h] According to OEF/OIF/OND Care Management Program officials, servicemembers and veterans are either referred to the program by a military treatment facility or are screened into the program when a servicemember or veteran initially seeks VA services at a VA treatment facility.

FRCP

The FRCP was established in January 2008. Developed as a joint program by DOD and VA, but administered by VA, the program was designed to provide care coordination services to servicemembers and veterans who were "severely" wounded, ill, and injured after September 11, 2001. (See table 13.)

Table 13. Federal Recovery Coordination Program (FRCP) Enrollment Populations and Characteristics, Fiscal Years 2008 through 2011

	Fiscal year			
	2008	*2009*	*2010*	*2011*
Program enrollment for the FRCP				
Total enrollment	*177*	*522*	*823*	*1,022*
Servicemembers	132	325	394	573
National Guard[a]	11	51	84	87
Reservists[a]	7	30	45	63
Veterans	43	194	429	449
Others	2	3	0	0
Population characteristics				
Enrollees with combat-related conditions	ND	ND	ND	ND
Enrollees with non-combat-related conditions	ND	ND	ND	ND

	Fiscal year			
	2008	*2009*	*2010*	*2011*
Enrollees with conditions not classified as either combat- or non-combat-related	ND	ND	ND	ND
Referrals and assists				
Total number of servicemembers referred to the program	*179*	*257*	*268*	*362*
Servicemembers referred and enrolled in the program	132	194	222	293
Servicemembers referred and assisted, but not enrolled in the program	ND	ND	ND	ND
Servicemembers referred but not enrolled in or assisted by the program	47	63	46	68
Total number of veterans referred to the program	*44*	*171*	*165*	*119*
Veterans referred and enrolled in the program	43	155	150	66
Veterans referred and assisted, but not enrolled in the program	ND	ND	ND	ND
Veterans referred but not enrolled in or assisted by the program	1	16	15	53

Legend: ND indicates that no data are available.

Source: GAO analysis of FRCP data.

[a]According to an FRCP official, the total number of servicemembers who are active duty cannot be delineated because the National Guard and Reservist numbers are descriptive data points and do not designate whether the enrollee is active duty or veteran. In addition, not all National Guard and Reservists are included in the data due to database limitations that have since been resolved.

The program uses federal recovery coordinators to monitor and coordinate clinical services, including facilitating and coordinating medical appointments, and nonclinical services, such as providing assistance with obtaining financial benefits or special accommodations, needed by program enrollees and their families. Federal recovery coordinators serve as the single point of contact among all of the case managers of DOD, VA, and other governmental and private case management programs that provide services directly to servicemembers and veterans.

Referral Information Tracked by DOD and VA Case Management and Care Coordination Programs

DOD and VA case management and care coordination programs primarily identify servicemembers and veterans who may be eligible for enrollment through referrals. Tracking referral information, including the number of those who were referred and enrolled or not enrolled in the program, may indicate whether the programs are identifying those who could benefit from their services. However, fewer than half of the DOD and VA case management and care coordination programs that we reviewed track this type of referral information. (See table 14.)

Table 14. Referral Information Routinely Tracked by DOD and VA Case Management and Care Coordination Programs

Program	Referral information routinely tracked	Types of referral information tracked, if any
Army		
Army Warrior Care and Transition Program: Warrior Transition Units and Community-Based Warrior Transition Units	√	Referral sources for program enrollees
Army Warrior Care and Transition Program: Army Wounded Warrior Program	√	Total number of referrals made to the program Number of those referred to the program who were enrolled into the program Number of those referred to the program who were enrolled and provided short-term assistance by the program, but who were later found ineligible for the program and disenrolled Number of those referred to the program who were not enrolled into the program
Navy/Coast Guard		
Navy Safe Harbor Program	√[a]	Total number of referrals made to the program Number of those referred to the program who were enrolled into the program Number of those referred to the program who were provided short-term assistance by the program, but not enrolled Number of those referred to the program who were not enrolled into the program or provided short-term assistance by the program
Air Force		
Air Force Wounded Warrior Program		According to Air Force Wounded Warrior Program officials, since the program only serves servicemembers with combat-related conditions, most

Program	Referral information routinely tracked	Types of referral information tracked, if any
		referrals come from casualty reports and the disability evaluation process, where it is determined whether a servicemember's wound, illness, or injury is combatrelated.
Air Force Recovery Care Program		None
Marine Corps		
Marine Corps Wounded Warrior Regiment		According to a Marine Corps Wounded Warrior Regiment official, although a policy exists requiring referral information to be collected, the policy was not always enforced.[b]
United States Special Operations Command		
United States Special Operations Command's Care Coalition		According to a United States Special Operations Command's Care Coalition official, the program does not track referral information because there is no field in its database to track this information. However, according to this official, the program is able to access this information from the individual military services.
Department of Veterans Affairs		
Operation Enduring Freedom/Operation Iraqi Freedom/Operation New Dawn Care Management Program	√	Total number of referrals made to the program from military treatment facilities
Federal Recovery Coordination Program	√	Total number of referrals made to the program Number of those referred to the program who were enrolled into the program Number of those referred to the program who were provided short-term assistance by the program, but not enrolled Number of those referred to the program who are not enrolled into the program or provided short-term assistance by the program

Source: GAO analysis of DOD and VA data.

[a] According to a Navy Safe Harbor Program official, the database used to track referral information did not capture accurate data until it was upgraded in 2010.

[b] According to a Marine Corps Wounded Warrior Program official, as of fiscal year 2012, data on referral information are routinely collected.

APPENDIX II. MEDICAL CATEGORY ASSIGNMENT PROCESS FOR CARE COORDINATION PROGRAMS

The Senior Oversight Committee intended for the Federal Recovery Coordination Program (FRCP) and the Recovery Coordination Program (RCP) to be complementary programs, specifically identifying which population of wounded, ill, and injured servicemembers would be assigned to the two programs.

On the basis of work done for the committee, the Department of Defense (DOD) sent a report to congressional committees in 2008 outlining a medical category assignment process based on the severity of each servicemember's medical condition, along with input from the servicemember and his or her unit commander, to determine whether servicemembers would be directed either to the FRCP or to the RCP programs for care coordination services.

In concept, the medical category assignment process would have resulted in wounded, injured, or ill servicemembers being assigned to one of three categories. Servicemembers designated as Category 1 were those who were found to have *mild* injury or illness, who were expected to return to duty in less than 180 days of medical treatment, and primarily received local outpatient and short-term inpatient treatment and rehabilitation.

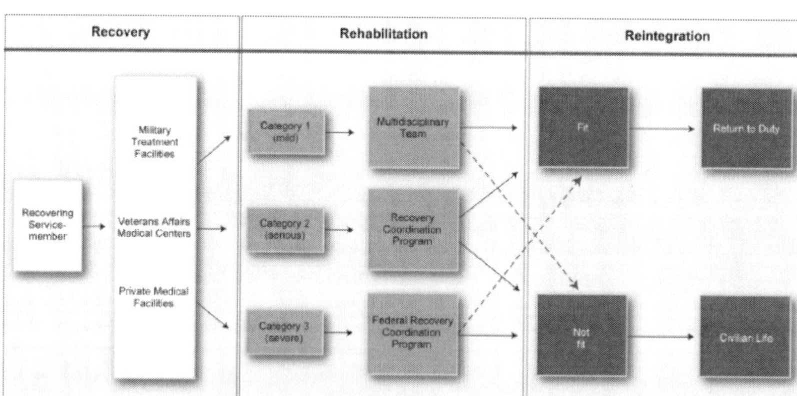

Note: In this figure, solid arrows indicate typical or expected results and dashed arrows indicate alternative, but possible, outcomes.

Figure 3. The Department of Defense's Vision of the Assignment Process for the Recovery Coordination Program and the Federal Recovery Coordination Program.

Servicemembers designated as Category 2 were those with *serious* injury or illness, who were unlikely to return to duty in less than 180 days, and may be medically separated from the military.[1] Servicemembers designated as Category 3 were those with *severe* injury or illness, who were highly unlikely to return to duty, and were most likely to be medically separated from the military. The category designation was intended to be used to determine whether the recovering servicemember was subsequently referred to a care coordination program, in that Category 1 servicemembers would not be referred to a care coordination program, unless their medical or psychological conditions worsen; Category 2 servicemembers would be referred to the RCP; and Category 3 servicemembers would be referred to the FRCP. (See figure 3.)

RELATED GAO PRODUCTS

Military Disability System: Improved Monitoring Needed to Better Track and Manage Performance. GAO-12-676. Washington, D.C.: August 28, 2012.

Military Disability System: Preliminary Observations on Efforts to Improve Performance. GAO-12-718T. Washington, D.C.: May 23, 2012.

More Efficient and Effective Government: Opportunities to Reduce Duplication, Overlap and Fragmentation, Achieve Savings, and Enhance Revenue. GAO-12-449T. Washington, D.C.: February 28, 2012.

2012 Annual Report: Opportunities to Reduce Duplication, Overlap and Fragmentation, Achieve Savings, and Enhance Revenue. GAO-12-342SP. Washington, D.C.: February 28, 2012.

DOD and VA Health Care: Action Needed to Strengthen Integration across Care Coordination and Case Management Programs. GAO-12-129T. Washington, D.C.: October 6, 2011.

VA and DOD Health Care: First Federal Health Care Center Established, but Implementation Concerns Need to Be Addressed. GAO-11-570. Washington, D.C.: July 19, 2011.

Federal Recovery Coordination Program: Enrollment, Staffing, and Care Coordination Pose Significant Challenges. GAO-11-572T. Washington, D.C.: May 13, 2011.

Information Technology: Department of Veterans Affairs Faces Ongoing Management Challenges. GAO-11-663T. Washington, D.C.: May 11, 2011.

Military and Veterans Disability System: Worldwide Deployment of Integrated System Warrants Careful Monitoring. GAO-11-633T. Washington, D.C.: May 4, 2011.

DOD and VA Health Care: Federal Recovery Coordination Program Continues to Expand but Faces Significant Challenges. GAO-11-250. Washington, D.C.: March 23, 2011.

Electronic Health Records: DOD and VA Should Remove Barriers and Improve Efforts to Meet Their Common System Needs. GAO-11-265.
Washington, D.C.: February 2, 2011.

End Notes

[1] "Soldiers Face Neglect, Frustration at Army's Top Medical Facility," Washington Post (Washington, D.C.: Feb. 18, 2007); "The Other Walter Reed: The Hotel Aftermath," Washington Post (Washington, D.C.: Feb. 19, 2007); and "Hospital Investigates Former Aid Chief," Washington Post (Washington, D.C.: Feb. 20, 2007).

[2] Independent Review Group, Rebuilding the Trust: Report on Rehabilitative Care and Administrative Processes at Walter Reed Army Medical Center and National Naval Medical Center (Arlington, Va.: April 2007); Task Force on Returning Global War on Terror Heroes, Report to the President (April 2007); President's Commission on Care for America's Returning Wounded Warriors, Serve, Support, Simplify (July 2007); Veterans' Disability Benefits Commission, Honoring the Call to Duty: Veterans' Disability Benefits in the 21st Century (October 2007); and Department of Defense Office of the Inspector General, Department of Veterans Affairs Office of the Inspector General, DOD/VA Care Transition Process for Service Members Injured in OIF/OEF (June 2008).

[3] According to the Case Management Society of America, case management is defined as a collaborative process of assessment, planning, facilitation, and advocacy for options and services to meet an individual's health needs through communication and available resources to promote high quality, cost-effective outcomes.

[4] See list of related GAO products at the end of this report.

[5] In this report, we will use the term "recovering servicemembers" to denote wounded, ill, and injured servicemembers.

[6] Pub. L. No. 110-181, § 1611, 122 Stat. 3, 433 (2008).

[7] National Defense Authorization Act for Fiscal Year 2010, Pub. L. No. 111-84, § 724, 123 Stat. 2190, 2389 (2009).

[8] Department of Defense Task Force on the Care, Management, and Transition of Recovering Wounded, Ill, and Injured Members of the Armed Forces, Department of Defense Recovering Warrior Task Force 2010-2011 Annual Report (September 2011).

[9] To understand how VA interacts with servicemembers, the Recovering Warrior Task Force reviewed VA programs, including those that assist servicemembers with the transition from DOD's to VA's health care system.

[10] According to the National Coalition on Care Coordination, care coordination is a client-centered, assessment-based interdisciplinary approach to integrating health care and social support services in which an individual's needs and preferences are assessed, a

comprehensive care plan is developed, and services are managed and monitored by an identified care coordinator.

[11] See Hearing on the Federal Recovery Coordination Program: From Concept to Reality, Subcommittee on Health, Committee on Veterans' Affairs, House of Representatives (May 13, 2011); and Review of the VA and DOD Integrated Disability Evaluation System, Hearing before the Committee on Veterans' Affairs, United States Senate (Nov. 18, 2010).

[12] Pub. L. No. 110-181, § 1615(d), 122 Stat. 2, 447.

[13] GAO has produced a body of work assessing progress made to improve care, management, and transition of recovering servicemembers, including: Recovering Servicemembers: DOD and VA Have Made Progress to Jointly Develop Required Polices but Additional Challenges Remain, GAO-09-540T (Washington, D.C.: Apr. 29, 2009); Recovering Servicemembers: DOD and VA Have Jointly Developed the Majority of Required Policies but Challenges Remain, GAO-09-728 (Washington, D.C.: July 8, 2009); DOD and VA Health Care: Federal Recovery Coordination Program Continues to Expand but Faces Significant Challenges, GAO-11-250 (Washington, D.C.: Mar. 23, 2011); DOD and VA Health Care: Action Needed to Strengthen Integration across Care Coordination and Case Management Programs, GAO-12-129T (Washington, D.C.: Oct. 6, 2011).

[14] We selected key care coordination and case management programs that provide assistance to recovering servicemembers and veterans—many of which were created or modified after Walter Reed media reports. These programs have also been the subject of prior reviews by GAO and others.

[15] See list of related GAO products.

[16] The terms "wounded, ill, and injured" are used by DOD and VA as general classifications of servicemembers or veterans with regard to their medical condition. "Wounded" generally means any injury inflicted by an external force during combat. "Ill and injured" refers to any illness or injury in the line of duty that may render the servicemember medically unfit to perform the duties of his or her office, grade, rank, or rating.

[17] President's Commission on Care for America's Returning Wounded Warriors, Serve, Support, Simplify.

[18] OEF, which began in October 2001, supports combat operations in Afghanistan and other locations, and OIF, which began in March 2003, supports combat operations in Iraq and other locations. Since September 1, 2010, OIF is referred to as Operation New Dawn (OND).

[19] Federal Recovery Coordinators are intended to coordinate all care and benefits for their enrollees, including coordinating assistance from private sector programs.

[20] Pub. L. No. 110-181, § 1635, 122 Stat. 3, 460-63.

[21] Interoperability is the ability of two or more systems or components to exchange information and to use the information that has been exchanged.

[22] Recovering servicemembers include those who are wounded, ill, or injured in a combat zone or due to an incident that occurred in the United States or overseas while in active status.

[23] According to a VA official, in fiscal year 2013, VA will hire 10 additional liaisons and expand the number of MTFs where liaisons will be located to 21.

[24] The VA OEF/OIF/OND Care Management Program screens all returning combat veterans to determine if case management services are required.

[25] Not all wounded, ill, and injured servicemembers and veterans are eligible for access to these programs. Most military service wounded warrior programs only serve those who are "seriously" and "severely" wounded, ill, and injured.

[26] Casualty reports, including personnel casualty reports, are electronic messages that contain casualty information including type of injury, where the injury occurred, and location of the injured servicemember.

[27] We found that referrals by unit command staff are most likely, because they have the most knowledge about servicemembers' conditions, injuries, and treatment locations.

[28] GAO-11-250.

[29] Servicemembers are eligible for certain VA benefits while still on active duty, including access to treatment at specialized VA facilities and grants for home and car modifications.

[30] Operation Warfighter is a DOD-sponsored internship program for wounded, ill, and injured servicemembers who are at MTFs. Operation Warfighter is designed to provide recuperating servicemembers with meaningful activity outside of the hospital environment that assists in their wellness and offers a formal means of transition back to the civilian workforce. Open to active duty, National Guard and Reserve components, Operation Warfighter represents an opportunity for servicemembers in a medical hold status to build their resumes, explore employment interests, develop job skills, and gain valuable work experience that will prepare them for the future (see www.militaryhomefront.dod.mil).

[31] The Warrior Athlete Reconditioning program provides recreational activities and competitive athletic opportunities to recovering servicemembers to improve their physical and mental quality of life throughout the continuum of recovery and transition. The program is designed to enhance recovery by engaging recovering servicemembers in physical and cognitive activities outside of traditional therapy settings.

[32] Servicemembers do not have to be enrolled in or attached to a wounded warrior program to participate in the VA Liaison for Healthcare Program or the Warrior Athlete Reconditioning Program.

[33] Recovering Warrior Task Force, Department of Defense Recovering Warrior Task Force 2010-2011 Annual Report.

[34] GAO, Military Disability System: Preliminary Observations on Efforts to Improve Performance, GAO-12-718T (Washington, D.C.: May 23, 2012). For additional information about IDES, see reports listed on the related products page.

[35] The fiscal year 2008 and 2011 averages include only those servicemembers who completed IDES and received VA benefits. The averages do not include other outcomes, such as servicemembers who were found fit and returned to duty. Not all reservists complete the VA benefit phase and thus DOD does not apply the 30-day goal for this phase to reservists. For those reservists who do go through the VA benefits phase, this time is reflected in the overall time in IDES.

[36] As we have previously testified, other reasons that could impact the increase in IDES processing times include large case loads and insufficient staff to complete a stage of IDES in a timely manner.

[37] Department of Defense Office of the Inspector General, Special Plans and Operations, Assessment of DOD Wounded Warrior Matters-Camp Lejeune (March 2012) and Department of Defense Office of the Inspector General, Special Plans and Operations, Assessment of DOD Wounded Warrior Matters-Wounded Warrior Battalion-West Headquarters and Southern California Units (August 2012).

[38] See, for example, GAO, Electronic Health Records: DOD and VA Efforts to Achieve Full Interoperability Are Ongoing; Program Office Management Needs Improvement, GAO-09-775 (Washington, D.C.: July 28, 2009); Electronic Health Records: DOD and VA Interoperability Efforts Are Ongoing; Program Office Needs to Implement Recommended Improvements, GAO-10-332 (Washington, D.C.: Jan. 28, 2010) and Electronic Health

Records: DOD and VA Should Remove Barriers and Improve Efforts to Meet Their Common System Needs, GAO-11-265 (Washington, D.C.: Feb. 2, 2011).

[39] DOD policy requires that, upon retirement, discharge, or end of active obligated service, records be transferred to the VA Records Management Center if the servicemember is not applying for VA benefits or the appropriate VA Regional Office if the servicemember has applied or plans to apply for VA benefits. Department of Defense, Service Treatment Record (STR) and Non-Service Treatment Record (NSTR) Life Cycle Management, DOD Instruction 6040.45, Enclosure 3, (Oct. 28, 2010). The transfer of records from DOD to a VA medical facility is achieved under different procedures.

[40] In 2008, DOD established the Office of Transition Policy and Care Coordination which was renamed the Office of Wounded Warrior Care and Transition Policy (WWCTP). Reporting to the Under Secretary of Defense for Personnel and Readiness, up until June 2012, WWCTP served as a single, centralized office for developing policy, coordinating interagency collaboration, and conducting outreach to address the broad set of issues confronted by wounded, ill and injured service members and their families. WWCTP also provided program oversight for the integrated disability evaluation system process and care coordination.

[41] The Joint Executive Council was established by law in November 2003 to provide senior leadership for collaboration and resource sharing between DOD and VA. Through a joint strategic planning process, the Joint Executive Council recommends to the Secretaries the strategic direction for the joint coordination and sharing efforts between the two departments and oversees the implementation of those efforts.

[42] With the change of presidential administration in January 2009, the Deputy Secretary of Defense and Deputy Secretary of Veterans Affairs were replaced.

[43] GAO-09-728.

[44] Department of Defense Task Force on the Care, Management, and Transition of Recovering Wounded, Ill, and Injured Members of the Armed Forces, Department of Defense Recovering Warrior Task Force 2011-2012 Annual Report (August 2012).

[45] Recovering Warrior Task Force, Department of Defense Recovering Warrior Task Force 2011-2012 Annual Report.

[46] Department of Defense, Recovery Coordination Program, DOD Instruction 1300.24, (Dec. 1, 2009).

[47] See GAO, Military and Veterans Disability System: Pilot Has Achieved Some Goals, but Further Planning and Monitoring Needed, GAO-11-69 (Washington, D.C.: Dec . 6, 2010); Military and Veterans Disability System: Worldwide Deployment of Integrated System Warrants Careful Monitoring, GAO-11-633T (Washington, D.C.: May 4, 2011); and GAO-12-718T.

[48] See Pub. L. No. 111-84, § 906, 123 Stat. 2190, 2425 (2009).

[49] Recovering Warrior Task Force, Department of Defense Recovering Warrior Task Force 2010-2011 Annual Report.

[50] Recovering Warrior Task Force, Department of Defense Recovering Warrior Task Force 2011-2012 Annual Report.

[51] See GAO-11-69; GAO-11-633T; GAO-12-718T; Electronic Health Records: DOD and VA Have Increased Their Sharing of Health Information, but More Work Remains, GAO-08-954 (Washington, D.C.: July 28, 2008); Electronic Health Records: DOD's and VA's Sharing of Information Could Benefit from Improved Management, GAO-09-268 (Washington, D.C.: Jan. 28, 2009); Information Technology: Challenges Remain for VA's

Sharing of Electronic Health Records with DOD, GAO-09-427T (Washington, D.C.: Mar. 12, 2009); GAO-09-775; and GAO-10-332.

[52] GAO-11-69.

[53] GAO-12-718T.

[54] Veterans Opportunity to Work (VOW) to Hire Heroes Act, Pub. L. No. 112-56, tit. II, 125 Stat. 712 (2011).

[55] GAO, Military System: Improved Monitoring Needed to Better Track and Manage Performance. GAO-12-676 (Washington, D.C.: Aug. 28, 2012).

[56] See Pub. L. No. 110-181, § 1635, 122 Stat. 3, 460-63 (2008).

[57] Legislative Hearing on H.R. 2383, H.R. 2388, H.R. 2243 and H.R. 2470, Before the Subcommittee on Oversight and Investigations of the Committee on Veterans Affairs, 112th Cong. (July 20, 2011) (statement of Debra M. Filippi, former Director, U.S. Department of Defense/U.S. Department of Veterans Affairs Interagency Program Office).

[58] As we reported in 2008, the Interagency Program Office was in the process of recruiting about 30 permanent staff members (see GAO-08-954).

[59] According to DOD and VA officials, the departments have identified 54 joint capabilities that will be implemented by the end of fiscal year 2017.

[60] GAO-12-129T.

[61] The Recovery Warrior Task Force also reported that DOD has partially addressed an additional 6 recommendations and noted that 13 recommendations remain open.

[62] Responding to a recommendation of a consulting firm that advised VA on its care coordination and case management policy, the VA Chief of Staff directed that VA conduct a department-wide inventory and review of its existing care coordination and case management programs and personnel.

[63] Communities of practice are groups of people who engage, through regular interaction with one another, in a process of collective learning in a shared domain of human endeavor.

[64] The Joint Executive Council meets on a bimonthly basis.

End Notes for Appendix I

[1] According to the National Coalition on Care Coordination, care coordination is a client-centered, assessment-based interdisciplinary approach to integrating health care and social support services in which an individual's needs and preferences are assessed, a comprehensive care plan is developed, and services are managed and monitored by an identified care coordinator.

[2] According to the Case Management Society of America, case management is defined as a collaborative process of assessment, planning, facilitation, and advocacy for options and services to meet an individual's health needs through communication and available resources to promote high quality, cost-effective outcomes.

[3] Military services operate multiple programs that are specialized to serve different populations, such as the severely wounded or surviving family members. For example, within the Air Force's Warrior and Survivor Care Program, the Air Force operates three distinct programs: (1) the Air Force Wounded Warrior Program to serve those who were injured in combat; (2) the Air Force Recovery Care Program to serve other seriously and severely wounded, ill, and injured; and (3) the Air Force Survivor Assistance Program, to serve surviving family members or caregivers of wounded, ill, and injured servicemembers.

[4] For the purpose of this appendix we will be discussing seven of the case management and care coordination programs established by the military services to assist recovering servicemembers and veterans with recovery, rehabilitation, and transition either back to military service or to civilian life.

[5] DOD defines command and control as the exercise of authority and direction by a properly designated commander over assigned and attached forces in the accomplishment of the mission.

[6] The program was originally named the Army Medical Action Plan.

[7] Warrior Transition Units are technically an Army brigade, battalion, or company that provides command and control, administrative support, primary care and case management and other services to promote readiness of soldiers and family to transition back to active duty or to civilian life. For the purposes of this report, we are categorizing it as a wounded warrior program.

[8] The Community-based Warrior Transition Unit Program allows servicemembers to live at home and perform duty at a location near home while receiving medical care.

[9] Warrior transition units and community-based warrior transition units serve Active Component servicemembers as well as servicemembers in National Guard and Reserve Components, but do not serve veterans.

[10] The Army Wounded Warrior Program was originally named the Disabled Soldier Support System.

[11] According to Navy Safe Harbor Program officials, the program evolved from the Navy's preexisting Military Severely Injured Center & Casualty Office.

[12] The Air Force Warrior and Survivor Care Program's Survivor Assistance Program primarily provides services to the families of wounded, ill, and injured servicemembers.

[13] District Injured Support Coordinators may also provide support to Reserve and Active Duty Marines in remote locations away from military or other federal resources.

[14] In addition, the Department of Veterans Affairs operates other dedicated programs and systems of care including Polytrauma/Traumatic Brain Injury, Spinal Cord Injury and Diseases, Visual Impairment, and Mental Health that provide specialized lifelong clinical care and care management for these special cohorts of veterans.

End Note for Appendix II

[1] DOD subsequently modified the 180-day criteria to "within a time specified by his or her military department" to accommodate different standards used by the Marine Corps and the Army.

In: Recovering Servicemembers and Veterans ISBN: 978-1-62417-775-0
Editors: Ira Wachtel and Gina Nutting

Chapter 2

MILITARY DISABILITY SYSTEM: IMPROVED MONITORING NEEDED TO BETTER TRACK AND MANAGE PERFORMANCE*

United States Government Accountability Office

ABBREVIATIONS

DOD	Department of Defense
IDES	integrated disability evaluation system
MEB	medical evaluation board
PEB	physical evaluation board
VA	Department of Veterans Affairs
VTA	Veterans Tracking Application
WCP	Office of Warrior Care Policy
WWCTP	Office of Wounded Warrior Care & Transition Policy

* This is an edited, reformatted and augmented version of The United States Government Accountability Office publication, Report to Congressional Committees, GAO-12-676, dated August 2012.

Why GAO Did This Study

Since 2007, DOD and VA have jointly operated IDES—which is intended to expedite benefits for injured servicemembers. IDES replaced the departments' separate processes for evaluating servicemembers for fitness and disability. Initially a pilot at 3 military treatment facilities, IDES is now in place at military treatment facilities worldwide. In previous reports, GAO identified a number of challenges as IDES expanded to more facilities, including staffing shortages and difficultly meeting timeliness goals.

In light of IDES' expansion, GAO was asked to examine: (1) the extent to which DOD and VA are meeting IDES timeliness and servicemember satisfaction performance goals, and (2) steps the agencies are taking to improve IDES performance. GAO analyzed IDES timeliness and customer satisfaction data, visited six IDES sites with varying performance, and interviewed DOD and VA officials.

What GAO Recommends

To improve monitoring of IDES timeliness and satisfaction, GAO recommends that DOD and VA work together to (1) develop plans for completing the ongoing business process review and implementing any resulting recommendations and (2) improve the accuracy of case information at the point of data entry; and that (3) DOD consider alternative approaches to measuring satisfaction. DOD and VA concurred with GAO's recommendations.

What GAO Found

Case processing times under the Integrated Disability Evaluation System (IDES) have increased over time, and measures of servicemember satisfaction have shortcomings. Since 2008, annual average processing times for IDES cases have steadily climbed, while the percentage of cases meeting established timeliness goals declined. Average case processing times reached 394 and 420 days for active and reserve component members in fiscal year 2011—compared to goals of 295 and 305 days, respectively, and just 19 percent of active duty and 18 percent of guard or reserve servicemembers completed the process and received benefits within established goals. Of the four phases comprising IDES, the medical evaluation board phase increasingly fell short of timeliness goals, while the physical evaluation board phase, although meeting goals, was taking increasingly more time to complete. With respect to servicemember satisfaction with the IDES process, GAO found shortcomings in how these data are collected and reported, such as unduly limiting who is eligible to receive a survey and computing average satisfaction scores in a manner that may overstate them. Department of Defense (DOD) officials told GAO they are considering alternatives for gauging satisfaction with the process.

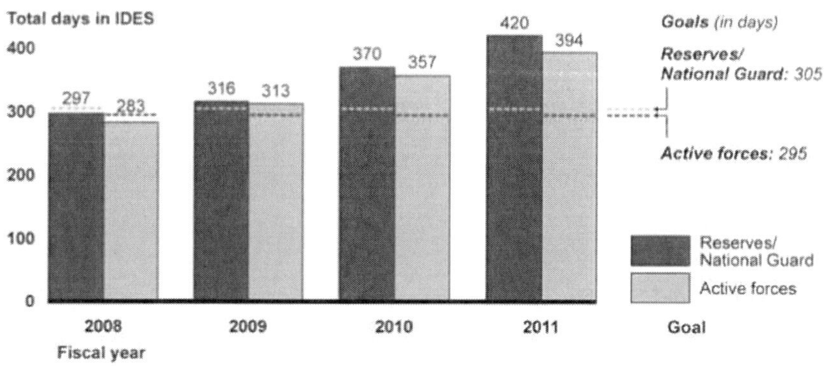

Source: GAO analysis of DOD and VA data.

Timeliness for IDES Cases Resulting in VA Benefits (by year case completed).

DOD and Veterans Affairs (VA) are taking steps to improve IDES performance, but progress to date is uneven and it is too early to assess their overall impact. For example, VA increased resources for completing exams and disability ratings while the Army is hiring additional staff for its medical evaluation boards. VA has met exam timeliness goals in the past several months, but other resources have yet to translate into lower processing times. DOD and VA are pursuing system upgrades so that staff and managers at IDES facilities can better track and manage the progress of servicemembers' cases. IDES officials have been working with the military services to correct case data that were inaccurately entered into VA's IDES tracking system, but have not yet identified a permanent solution to improve the accuracy of data input. Finally, DOD, with VA's assistance, is in the early stages of an in-depth review of the entire IDES process and its supporting IT systems. This effort is intended to improve understanding of how each step contributes to overall processing times and identify opportunities to streamline the process and supporting systems. However, timeframes for completing the review or issuing recommendations have yet to be established.

August 28, 2012

The Honorable Patty Murray
Chairman

The Honorable Richard Burr
Ranking Member
Committee on Veterans' Affairs
United States Senate

The Honorable Joseph I. Lieberman
Chairman
The Honorable Susan M. Collins
Ranking Member
Committee on Homeland Security and Governmental Affairs
United States Senate

Servicemembers who are injured in war or as the result of accidents and illnesses may face a difficult transition as they leave the military and become veterans. In response to concerns that wounded, ill, or injured servicemembers had to undergo two complex disability evaluations—first by the Department of Defense (DOD) then by the Department of Veterans Affairs (VA)—DOD and VA jointly designed a new integrated disability evaluation process to expedite the delivery of benefits to servicemembers. In November 2007, DOD and VA began pilot testing the integrated disability evaluation system (IDES) at three military treatment facilities in the Washington, D.C. area, and expanded the number of sites over time. As of October 1, 2011, IDES had replaced the military services' existing—or "legacy"—disability evaluation systems for almost all new disability cases.

Past GAO work highlighted challenges DOD and VA experienced while piloting the IDES and recommended a number of improvements. For instance, we reported in December 2010[1] that insufficient staff and logistical challenges contributed to delays in completing IDES cases and recommended the agencies take steps to ensure adequate staffing levels and develop a systematic process for monitoring caseloads. In response to ongoing concerns with IDES performance, this report provides information on (1) the extent to which DOD and VA are meeting IDES performance goals, and (2) steps DOD and VA are taking to improve IDES performance.

In conducting our work, we obtained DOD timeliness and customer satisfaction data from the inception of IDES in 2007 to December 2011. We assessed the reliability of these data and analyzed them to look for changes in performance over time; factors that may help or hinder performance; and relationships between servicemember satisfaction and case outcomes and timeliness. We supplemented these analyses with site visits to six military treatment facilities, where we spoke with DOD and VA staff as well as some servicemembers involved in the IDES process.[2] We selected these facilities to obtain perspectives from sites in different military services and geographical regions and with varying caseloads and performance outcomes. For both research objectives, we interviewed key officials involved with IDES at DOD, VA, and each of the military services, and reviewed pertinent reports, guidance, plans, relevant federal laws, regulations, directives, and other documents. We conducted this performance audit from May 2011 to August 2012, in accordance with generally accepted government auditing standards. These standards require that we plan and perform the audit to obtain sufficient, appropriate evidence to provide a reasonable basis for our findings and conclusions based on our audit objectives. We believe the evidence obtained provides a reasonable basis for our findings and conclusions based on our audit objectives.

BACKGROUND

The Disability Evaluation Process

The IDES process begins at a military treatment facility when a physician identifies one or more conditions that may interfere with a servicemember's ability to perform his or her duties.[3] The process involves four main phases: the Medical Evaluation Board (MEB), the Physical Evaluation Board (PEB), transition out of military service (transition), and VA benefits.

MEB phase: In this phase, medical examinations are conducted and decisions are made by the MEB regarding a servicemember's ability to continue to serve in the military. This phase involves four stages: (1) the servicemember is counseled by a DOD board liaison on what to expect during the IDES process; (2) the servicemember is counseled by a VA case manager on what to expect during the IDES process and medical exams are scheduled;[4] (3) medical exams are conducted according to VA standards for exams for disability compensation by VA, DOD, or contractor physicians, and (4) exam results are used by the MEB to identify conditions that limit the servicemember's ability to serve in the military.[5] Also during this stage, a servicemember can seek a rebuttal, or an impartial medical review by a physician not on the MEB, or both.

PEB phase: In this subsequent phase, decisions are made about the servicemember's fitness for duty, disability rating and DOD and VA disability benefits, and the servicemember has opportunities to appeal those decisions. This includes: (1) the informal PEB stage, an administrative review of the case file by the relevant military branch's PEB without the presence of the servicemember; (2) VA rating stage, where a VA rating specialist prepares a rating that covers the conditions that DOD determined made a servicemember unfit for duty and any other conditions claimed by the servicemember to VA.[6] This rating is prepared for use by both agencies in determining disability benefits. In addition, servicemembers have several opportunities to appeal different aspects of their disability evaluations: a servicemember dissatisfied with the decision on whether he or she is fit for duty may request a hearing with a "formal" PEB; a servicemember who disagrees with the formal PEB fitness decision can, under certain conditions, appeal to the reviewing authority of the PEB;[7] and a servicemember can ask for VA to reconsider its rating, but only for conditions found unfitting by the PEB.

Transition phase: If the servicemember is found unfit to serve, he or she enters the transition phase and begins the process of separating from the military. During this time, the servicemember may take accrued leave. Also, DOD board liaisons and VA case managers provide counseling on available benefits and services, such as job assistance.*VA benefits phase*: A servicemember found unfit and separated from service becomes a veteran and enters the VA benefits phase. VA finalizes its disability rating after receiving evidence of the servicemember's separation from military service. VA then starts to award monthly disability compensation to the veteran.

DOD and VA established timeliness goals for the IDES process to provide VA benefits to active duty servicemembers within 295 days of being referred into the process, and to reserve component members within 305 days (see figure 1). DOD and VA also established interim timeliness goals for each phase and stage of the IDES process. The overall timeframes are intended to represent an improvement over the legacy disability evaluation system, which was estimated to take 540 days to complete.

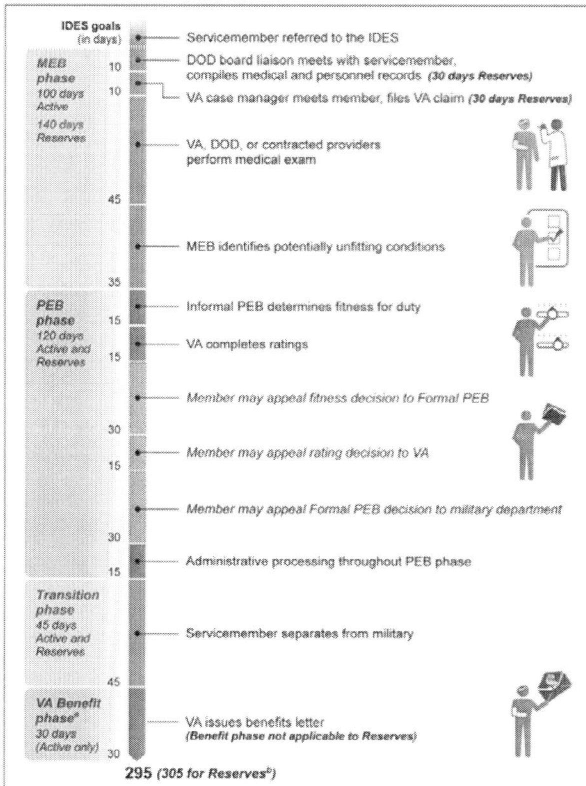

Source: GAO analysis of DOD and VA polices.

[a] Not all reservists complete the VA benefit phase and thus DOD does not apply the 30-day goal for this phase to reservists. For those reservists who do go through the VA benefits phase, this time is reflected in the overall time in IDES.

[b] DOD guidance allows 40 more days for reserve component members than for active duty members in completing the first two steps of the process, in order to provide sufficient time for employer notification, establish orders for active duty, and compile medical records. However, DOD and VA's goal for total IDES processing time is only 10 days longer for reserve component members than for active duty members because the VA benefit phase goal of 30 days is not applied to reserve component members.

Figure 1. Steps of the IDES Process and Timeliness Goals.

In addition to timeliness, the agencies also established a performance goal of having 80 percent of servicemembers satisfied with the IDES process. DOD measures satisfaction through surveys conducted after the completion of the

MEB, PEB, and transition phases. Each survey consists of approximately 30 questions, including 4 questions that ask about the servicemember's satisfaction with the overall IDES process up to that point. Reported satisfaction rates for each phase are based on an average of responses to these four questions, and reported overall satisfaction with IDES (which is used to track the percent satisfied under the performance goal) is an average of satisfaction rates for the three phases.

Rollout of IDES and Enrollment

From the original 3 pilot military treatment facilities in the Washington, D.C., area,[8] the IDES has expanded to 139 military treatment facilities in the U.S. and several other countries. DOD and VA first added 24 military treatment facilities to the pilot in fiscal years 2009 and 2010, bringing the pilot total to 27. In 2010, DOD and VA leadership decided to implement the IDES world-wide, and did so in 4 stages between October 2010 and September 2011, adding 112 military treatment facilities. As IDES expanded, the number of new cases enrolled in IDES has also increased, totaling 18,651 in fiscal year 2011 (see fig. 2). IDES caseloads vary by service, but the Army manages the bulk of IDES cases. Of new cases referred to IDES in fiscal year 2011, about 64 percent were in the Army, and much of the growth in caseload has been in the Army. Additionally, active duty servicemembers make up the majority of IDES cases, with about 88 percent of new cases in fiscal year 2011 involving this group (see figure 3).

IDES Processing Times Increased Over Time, While Measures of Servicemember Satisfaction Have Shortcomings

Overall IDES Case Processing Times Steadily Increased Since the Start of IDES

IDES timeliness has worsened since the inception of the program. Since fiscal year 2008, the average number of days for servicemember cases to be processed and receive benefits increased from 283 to 394 for active duty cases (compared to the goal of 295 days) and from 297 to 420, for reserve component cases (compared to the goal of 305 days) (see fig. 4).[9]

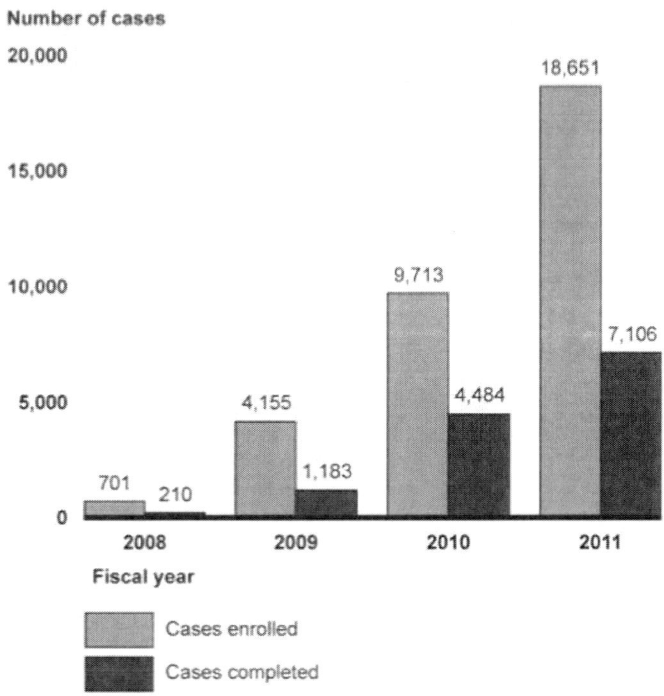

Source: GAO analysis of DOD and VA data.

Note: Cases completed include those who exited the IDES process, including those who received benefits or returned to duty.

Figure 2. IDES Cases Enrolled and Completed by Fiscal Year.

Along with increasing average processing times, the percent of IDES cases awarded benefits within timeliness goals has steadily declined. DOD's and VA's current goal is to complete 60 percent of IDES cases on time. In fiscal year 2008, an average of 63 percent of cases for active duty servicemembers and 65 percent for reservists completed the process and received benefits within the timeliness goals; by fiscal year 2011 this was down to 19 and 18 percent respectively (see figure 5). These trends also hold when considering all cases that completed the IDES process regardless of outcome, although overall processing times were shorter. (See app. III for more information on case processing times regardless of outcome.)

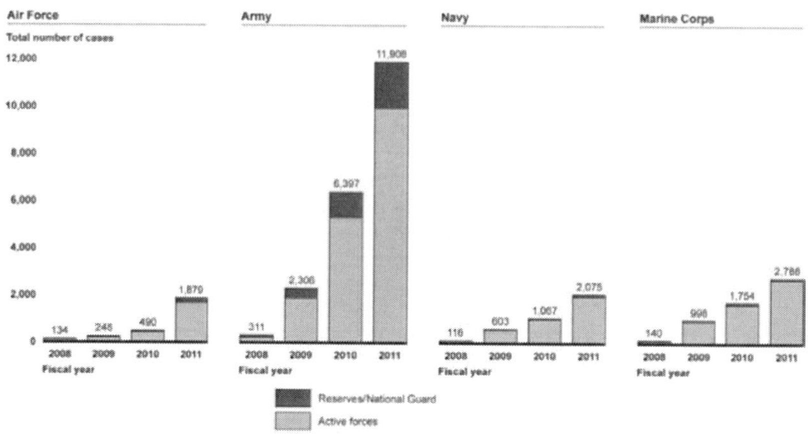

Source: GAO analysis of DOD and VA data.

Figure 3. Distribution of New IDES Cases Each Year by Military Service and Status.

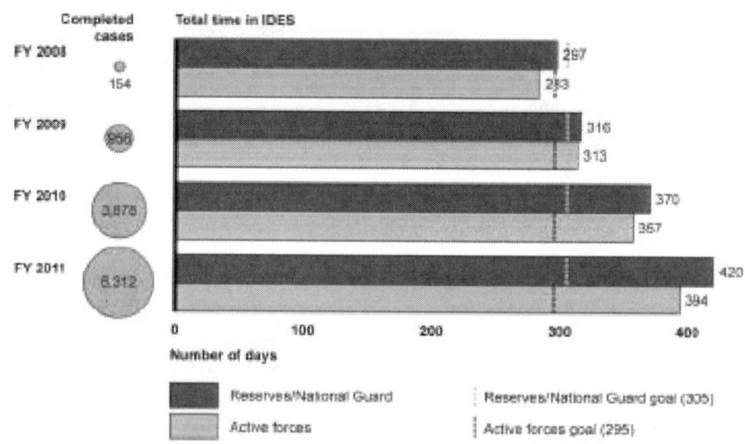

Source: GAO analysis of DOD and VA data.

Figure 4. Average Processing Times and Number of Completed Cases Resulting in Benefits by Fiscal Year of IDES Completion.

Key Contributors to Timeliness Problems Include Lengthy Medical Evaluations and Servicemember Separation Activities

When examining timeliness across the four phases that make up IDES, data show that average processing time regularly fell short of goals for three—

MEB, Transition, and VA Benefits. For example, for cases that completed the MEB phase in fiscal year 2011, active duty and reserve component members' cases took an average of 181 and 188 days respectively to be processed, compared to goals of 100 and 140 days. For the PEB phase, processing times increased over time, but were still within the established goal of 120 days. Along with increasing average processing times, the percentage of cases meeting goals for most phases has generally declined (see fig. 6). In particular, the MEB and Transition phases have lower percentages of cases meeting goals than the other phases in most years, especially for active duty cases.

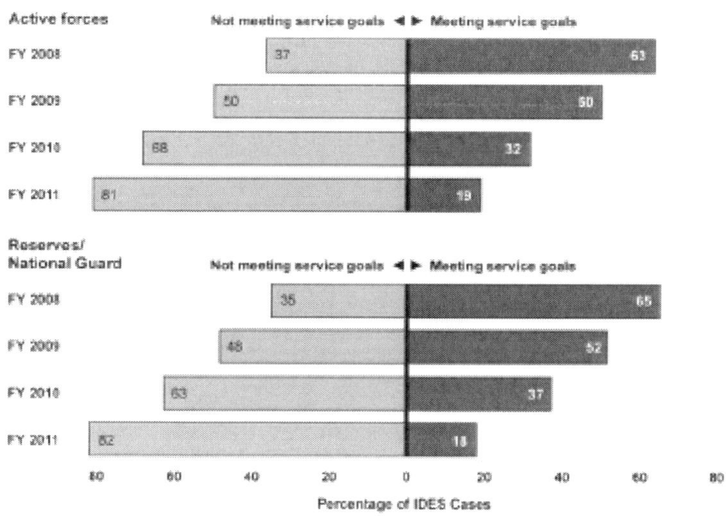

Source: GAO analysis of DOD and VA data.

Figure 5. Percentage of Cases Resulting in Benefits Meeting and Not Meeting Overall Processing Time Goals by Fiscal Year of IDES Completion.

MEB Phase

As noted above, the MEB phase was a key contributor to increases in overall processing times between 2008 and 2011 for both active duty servicemembers and reservists for cases that have completed the IDES process regardless of outcome (table 1). To obtain a better understanding of more recent timeliness trends within the MEB phase, GAO analyzed MEB timeliness of all cases—all fiscal years combined—that completed the MEB process by sorting them into two groups: (1) those that completed the entire IDES process, and (2) those that had not yet completed IDES but completed the MEB phase. As shown in figure 7, for the group that completed IDES, 30 percent of active duty servicemembers and 18 percent of reservists missed the goal by more than 90 days. For those still in IDES, representing more recent data, the picture is slightly better for active duty servicemembers with 37 percent of cases meeting the MEB goal and 25 percent missing the goal by more than 90 days. However, the percentage of reserve component members who missed the goal by more than 90 days increased from 18 to 28 percent.

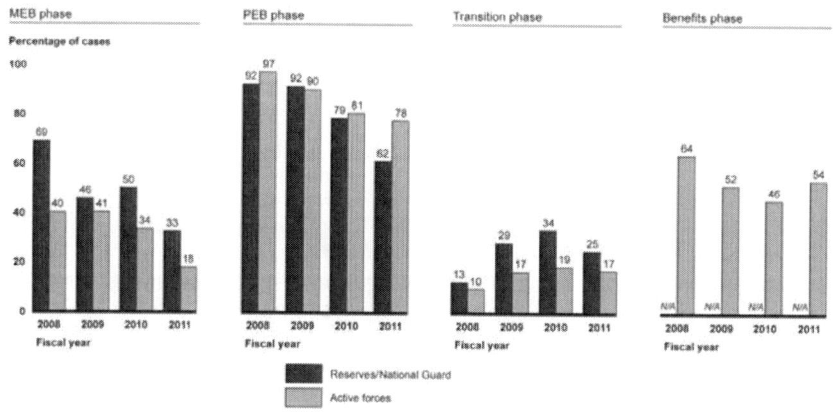

Source: GAO analysis of DOD and VA data.

Figure 6. Percent of Cases Meeting Timeliness Goals for each Phase of IDES by Fiscal Year of Completion.

Table 1. Average Processing Times for MEB Phase for Completed Cases by Fiscal Year of Completion (in days)

Component	Goal	FY 2008	FY2009	FY2010	FY2011
Active	100	114	126	141	181
Reserve	140	128	153	158	188

Source: GAO analysis of DOD and VA data.

For those servicemembers who were still enrolled in the MEB phase as of December 2011, the data show that 41 percent of active duty and 33 percent of reserve component servicemember cases had already missed the goal processing times (see fig. 8). Of these, 15 percent of active duty and 10 percent of reservist component servicemember cases missed the goal by more than 90 days.[10]

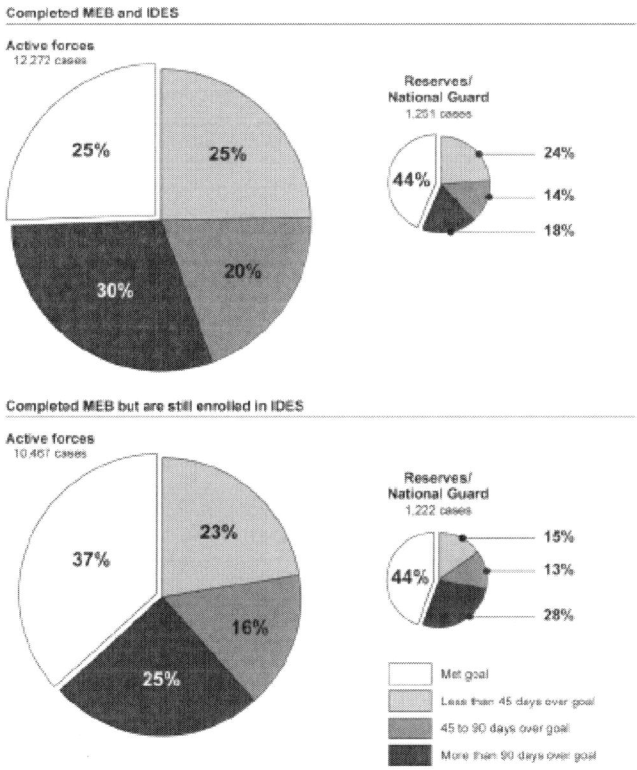

Source: GAO analysis of DOD and VA data.
Note: Numbers may not total 100 percent due to rounding.

Figure 7. Percent of Cases Completing MEB Within or in Excess of Goals All Fiscal Years Combined.

Within the MEB phase, significant delays have occurred in completing medical examinations (medical exam stage) and delivering an MEB decision (the MEB stage). For cases completing the MEB phase in fiscal year 2011, 31 percent of active duty and 29 percent of reservist cases met the 45-day goal for the medical exam stage and 20 percent of active duty and 17 percent of reservist cases met the 35-day goal for the MEB stage. Officials at some sites we visited told us that MEB phase goals were difficult to meet and not realistic given current resources.

For example:

- Some military officials noted that they did not have sufficient numbers of doctors to write the narrative summaries of exam results needed to complete the MEB stage in a timely manner.[11] One facility noted that while they have 7 doctors, they would need 11 additional doctors and 10 technician assistants to process cases through the initial medical exam and other additional disability specific examinations in a timely manner. Further, officials at another Army base we visited noted that there was a shortage of doctors and DOD board liaisons and that they had difficulty recruiting such staff due to the remote location of the base.
- At all the facilities we visited, officials told us DOD board liaisons and VA case managers had large case loads. While DOD has established a goal of 1 board liaison for every 20 servicemembers,[12] the ratios varied widely by military treatment facility with a range from 1:1 as the lowest to the highest of 1:75 according to recent data. Because of high case loads and a reported increase in the complexity of cases, staff at one facility reported a liaison to servicemember ratio of 1:80 and noted that liaisons must often prioritize cases to deal with the most pressing issues first. As a result, cases that might otherwise be quick to process take longer simply because they are waiting to be processed. Liaisons are often working overtime and weekends to keep up with cases.

Monthly data produced by DOD subsequent to the data we analyzed show significantly improved timeliness for the medical exam stage (66 percent of active duty cases met the goal in June 2012) and some improvement for the MEB stage (40 percent of active duty cases met the goal in the month of June 2012). However, it is too early to tell whether these improvements will continue going forward. (See app. III for DOD reported monthly data, October 2011 – June 2012[13] .)

PEB Phase

Since fiscal year 2008, the majority of cases have completed the PEB phase under the goal of 120 days, however, PEB timeliness has still worsened over time. In 2011, 78 percent of active duty and 62 percent of reservist cases that completed the entire IDES process met the PEB goal.

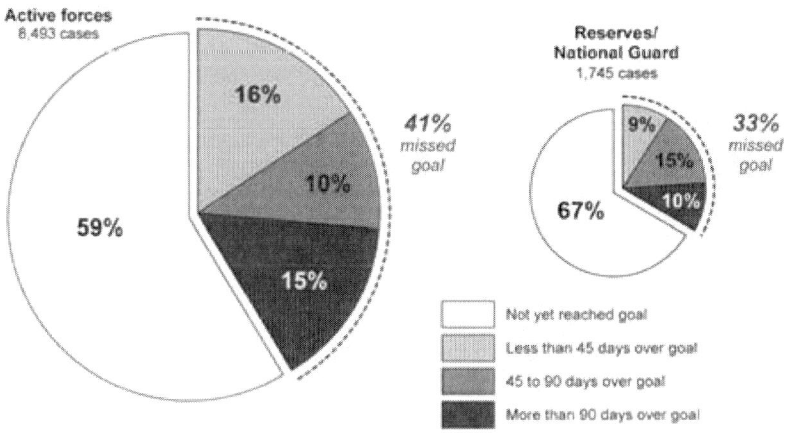

Source: GAO analysis of DOD and VA data.
Note: Numbers may not match numbers in the body of this report or total 100 percent due to rounding.

Figure 8. Timeliness of Cases Enrolled in MEB Stage as of December 2011.

Table 2. Average Processing Time in PEB Phase of IDES for Completed Cases (in days)

Component	Goal	FY 2008	FY2009	FY2010	FY2011
Active	120	42	58	80	93
Reserve	120	41	60	83	116

Source: GAO analysis of DOD and VA data.

The average processing time was 93 days for active duty servicemembers and 116 for reservists (see table 2).

Despite meeting the overall PEB goal in fiscal year 2011, established goals were not met for any of the interim PEB stages, including the informal PEB and VA rating stages which are the two stages all servicemembers must complete. For all cases that completed the PEB phase in fiscal year 2011, only 38 percent of active duty and 38 percent of reservists' cases received an informal PEB decision within the 15 days allotted. Further, only 32 percent of active duty and 27 percent of reservist cases received a preliminary VA rating within the 15-day goal. (see table 3).

Regarding delays with the VA rating, VA officials told us that staffing has been a challenge at their IDES rating sites and that this has slowed case processing. Monthly data produced by DOD subsequent to the data we analyzed show similar trends for the informal PEB and VA preliminary rating stages. As of June 2012 (most recent data available), active duty cases showed slight improvements in timeliness for the informal PEB stage (41 percent of cases meeting the goal and processing times averaging 24 days). The VA rating stage, on the other hand, showed slight declines in timeliness (31 percent of cases meeting the established goal and processing times of 35 days) relative to FY 2011 averages for active duty servicemembers. However, as noted before, it is too early to tell the extent to which such trends will continue. (See app. III for DOD reported monthly data, October – June 2012.)

Table 3. Average Processing Time for PEB Stages of IDES for Completed Cases (in days)

Stage of PEB Phase	Component	Goal	FY 2008	FY2009	FY2010	FY2011
Informal Physical Evaluation Board (IPEB)	Active	15	17	12	21	26
	Reserve	15	15	12	19	29
VA preliminary rating	Active	15	6	20	27	33
	Reserve	15	7	26	32	43
VA rating reconsideration[a]	Active	15	3	11	14	32
	Reserve	15	8	29	18	30
Formal Physical Evaluation Board (FPEB)[a]	Active	30	13	39	63	81
	Reserve	30	33	38	55	69
FPEB appeal[a]	Active	30	196	5	100	103
	Reserve	30	20	23	13	169

Source: GAO analysis of DOD and VA data

[a]These stages are appeals. Fewer servicemembers completed each of the appeal stages compared to the non-appeal stages, but the average days spent within the appeal stages generally and significantly surpassed the goal times.

Also during this phase, IDES planners allocated the majority of overall PEB processing time (75 out of the 120 days) for appeals—including a formal PEB hearing and a reconsideration of the VA ratings. According to officials, while the three appeal stages do not happen for every case, appeals can significantly increase processing times for any one case. However, only 20 percent of cases completed in fiscal year 2011 actually had any appeals; calling into question DOD and VA's assumption on the prevalence and average effect of appeals, and potentially masking processing delays in other mandatory parts of the PEB phase.

Transition Phase

The transition phase has consistently taken longer than its 45-day goal—almost twice as long on average. While processing times improved slightly for cases that completed this phase in fiscal year 2011 (from 79 days in fiscal year 2010 to 76 days in fiscal year 2011 for active duty cases), timeliness has remained consistently problematic since fiscal year 2008 (see table 4).

Table 4. Average Processing Time in Transition Phase of IDES for Completed Cases (in days)

Component	Goal	FY 2008	FY2009	FY2010	FY2011
Active	45	88	80	79	76
Reserve	45	81	73	82	75

Source: GAO analysis of DOD and VA data.

DOD lacks comprehensive data on how servicemembers spend their time in the transition phase, which includes many different activities related to separation from the military.

These activities vary widely depending on the case.[14] For example, during this phase servicemembers receive mandatory training such as job training through the Transition Assistance Program and may also receive counseling such as pre-discharge Vocational Rehabilitation and Employment counseling. In addition, servicemembers may be placed on temporary duty while house hunting, or to allow for a servicemember's children to complete the school year before moving.

Servicemembers may also take earned leave time—to which they are entitled—before separating from the service. For example, an Army official said that Army policy allows servicemembers to take up to 90 days of earned leave prior to separating, and that average leave time was about 80 days.

Because many of these activities can occur simultaneously or in small intermittent segments of time, DOD officials said it is difficult to track which activities servicemembers participate in or determine how much time each activity takes. DOD is exploring options for better tracking how time is spent in this phase.

Because a potentially substantial amount of the time in this phase may be for the personal benefit of servicemembers, DOD recently began reporting time in IDES with and without the transition phase included.

Benefits Phase

Processing time improved somewhat for the benefits phase (48 days in fiscal year 2010 to 38 days in fiscal year 2011), but continued to exceed the 30-day goal for active duty servicemembers (see table 5).[15]

Several factors may contribute to delays in this final phase. VA officials told us that cases cannot be closed without the proper discharge forms and that sometimes they do not receive this information in a timely manner from the military services. Additionally, if data are missing from the IDES tracking system (e.g., the servicemember already separated, but this was not recorded in the database), processing time will continue to accrue for cases that remain open in the system. Officials could not provide data on the extent to which these factors had an impact on processing times for pending cases, but said that once errors are detected and addressed, reported processing times are also corrected.

Table 5. Average Processing Time in Benefits Phase of IDES for Completed Cases (in days)

Component	Goal	FY 2008	FY2009	FY2010	FY2011
Active	30	29	43	48	38

Source: GAO analysis of DOD and VA data.

Shortcomings in the Design and Administration of Service Member Surveys Hamper their Usefulness

In addition to timeliness, DOD and VA evaluate IDES performance using the results of servicemember satisfaction surveys. In principle, all members have an opportunity to complete satisfaction surveys at the end of the MEB, PEB, and transition phases; however, under current survey procedures servicemembers become ineligible to complete a survey for either the PEB or transition phases if they did not complete a survey in an earlier phase. Additionally, servicemembers who start but do not complete a phase are not surveyed. As such, DOD may be missing opportunities to obtain input from servicemembers who did not complete a prior survey or exited IDES in the middle of a phase.[16] Further, response rates may be affected because DOD does not survey servicemembers once they separate from the service and become veterans. While it is not necessary for DOD to survey all servicemembers at the end of every phase,[17] the percentage and characteristics of servicemembers covered by the survey (i.e., who completed a phase and were ultimately interviewed) may be insufficient to establish that the survey results are representative of servicemember satisfaction, especially for later phases. (See table 6 for response and coverage rates.) DOD officials recently told us that they will consider alternative survey eligibility requirements, including working with the Office of Management and Budget for permission to interview veterans. (For additional information regarding the timing of the survey, see app. II).

In addition, alternate survey measures show lower satisfaction rates than those reported by DOD. Using DOD's measure, we found an overall satisfaction rate of about 67 percent since the inception of IDES. DOD defines a servicemember as satisfied if the average of his or her responses across several surveys is above 3 on a 5-point scale, with 3 denoting neither satisfied nor dissatisfied. However, using our alternate measure that defines servicemembers as satisfied only when all of their responses are 4 or above,[18] we calculated the satisfaction rate to be about 24 percent (see fig. 9).

Table 6. Survey Response and Coverage Rates

Phase	Service members who completed phase (N)	Service members eligible to be surveyed (i.e., completed both phase and survey for prior phase, if applicable)	Service members who completed survey	Response rate (Service members who completed survey ! Service members eligible)	Coverage rate (Servicemembers who completed survey ! Service members who completed phase)
MEB	25,212	all	9,604	38.1%	38.1%
PEB	18,296	8,968	4,795	53.5%	26.2%
Transition	12,352	3,996	2,893	72.4%	23.4%

Source: GAO analysis of DOD and VA data.

Our calculation is a more conservative measure of satisfaction, because it rules out the possibility that a servicemember is deemed "satisfied" even when he or she is dissatisfied on one or more questions in the scale. While not incorrect, DOD's scale can mask pockets of servicemember dissatisfaction. For example, an individual may indicate that he or she is very dissatisfied with one phase of the program, but satisfied with other phases, and the overall satisfaction score can be the same as one for a servicemember who is generally satisfied across all phases of the process. Measuring satisfaction, or even dissatisfaction, in different ways may provide a more complete picture of satisfaction and how it varies in different circumstances, and thus may reveal areas where DOD could focus on improving management and performance.

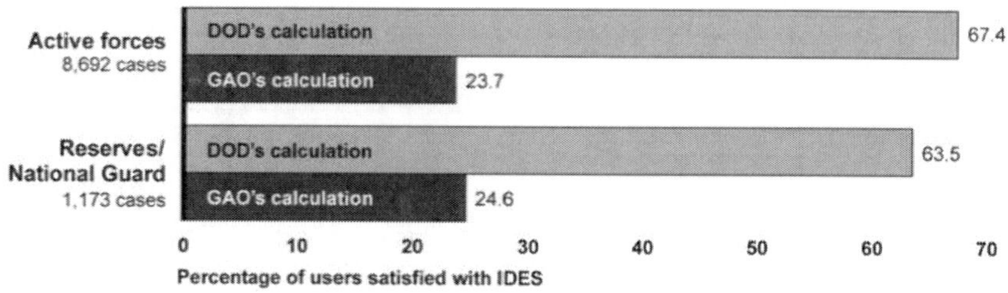

Source: GAO analysis of DOD and VA data.

Note: GAO combined reserve and national guard, while DOD reported satisfaction scores for guard and reserve separately.

Figure 9. Comparison of Percent of Servicemembers Satisfied Using GAO and DOD Calculations for Overall Satisfaction.

Finally, using either DOD's or our calculated measure, we found that overall satisfaction did not vary much according to differences in the experiences of servicemembers. For example, our model estimated that satisfaction varied by no more than approximately five percentage points across branch, component, disenrollment outcome, sex, MEB exam provider, enlisted and officer personnel classes, and the number of claimed and referred conditions. While lack of variation could be a positive outcome signaling consistent treatment, it could equally mean that the survey does not measure opinions in enough detail to discriminate among servicemembers' experiences.

Either way, such results provide little insight into identifying areas for improvement or effective practices. Further, while we found some association between servicemembers satisfaction and the timeliness of their case processing, we also found many servicemembers were highly dissatisfied even when their cases were completed on time, and many were highly satisfied even that PEB timeliness was "very poor" completed the phase on time, and 55 percent of those who said that MEB timeliness was "very good" did not complete on time. The lack of variation and/or correlation between satisfaction and experiences of servicemembers—coupled with low coverage rates—raise questions about the value of the survey results as a performance measure and program evaluation tool. (See app. II for more information on servicemember satisfaction results.)

DOD is reconsidering its options for measuring customer satisfaction, but has yet to select a particular approach. As noted above, possible changes might include widening the criteria for who is eligible for the survey, modifying survey questions, changing when and how the survey is delivered, and changing how satisfaction is calculated. Officials already concluded that the survey, in its current form, is not a useful management tool for determining what changes are needed in IDES and said that it is expensive to administer—costing approximately $4.3 million in total since the start of the IDES pilot. Navy officials told us they believed that the satisfaction surveys could be made more useful if they knew whether servicemember's satisfaction was actually influenced by the servicemember's desired or actual outcome of the IDES process. Further, Army officials already determined that the DOD survey is of limited value, and are proceeding with plans to field their own survey in the hopes of obtaining more detailed information at the facility level. Because of fiscal constraints, DOD suspended the survey in December 2011, but officials told us that they hope to resume collecting data in fiscal year 2013.

We identified two potential alternatives to assessing servicemember experiences.

- *Surveying a sample of servicemembers*: While a census gives each servicemember a chance to describe his or her experiences with IDES, DOD could collect the same data at a lower cost by surveying a probability sample of servicemembers. If appropriately designed and executed, a sample would accurately represent all groups of servicemembers and produce the necessary data for important subgroups, such as facilities or branches. Since the cost of administering a survey is strongly related to the number of people surveyed, probability sampling could also allow DOD to assess servicemember experiences while substantially reducing data collection costs.
- *Exit interviews*: In-depth interviews with servicemembers, completed at disenrollment from IDES, could also yield more detailed and actionable information about the program. Although the current survey includes open-ended questions, it is primarily designed to collect standardized, quantitative measures of satisfaction with broad aspects of IDES, such as fairness and the performance of DOD board liaisons and VA case managers. As a result, the survey provides a limited amount of detailed feedback on particular facilities, staff members, and stages of the process that managers might use to improve the servicemember experience, decrease processing times, or reduce cost. In contrast, semi-structured exit interviews would allow

servicemembers to provide this type of qualitative, detailed feedback. Interviewing servicemembers at the end of the process would also allow servicemembers to assess their overall experiences with IDES rather than at an earlier stage, without having completed the entire process. Exit interviews could also reach servicemembers who exit IDES without completing the process such as those who are returned to duty. Exit interviews, however, have the potential to be labor intensive and expensive.

RECENT ACTIONS AND ONGOING INITIATIVES MAY IMPROVE IDES PERFORMANCE, BUT IT IS TOO EARLY TO ASSESS THEIR OVERALL IMPACT

DOD and VA Took Steps to Address Previously Identified IDES Challenges

DOD and VA have undertaken a number of actions to address IDES challenges—many of which we identified in our past work. Some actions—such as increased oversight and staffing—represent important steps in the right direction, but progress is uneven in some areas.

Increased monitoring and oversight: We identified the need for agency leadership to provide continuous oversight of IDES in 2008[19] and the need for system-wide monitoring mechanisms in 2010. Since then, agency leadership has established mechanisms to improve communication, monitoring, and accountability.

- The secretaries of DOD and VA have met several times since February 2011 to discuss progress in improving IDES timeliness and have tasked their agencies to find ways to streamline the process so that the timeliness goals can be shortened. The secretaries also tasked their agencies to expand the use of expedited disability evaluations for severely combat-wounded servicemembers; [20] and develop a system to electronically transfer case files between DOD and VA locations.
- Senior Army and Navy officials regularly hold conferences to assess performance and address performance issues, including at specific facilities. With respect to the Army, meetings are led by the Army's vice-chief of staff and VA's chief of staff, and include reviews of

> performance where regional and local facility commanders provide feedback on best practices and challenges. For example, recent Army-VA conferences focused on delays in completion of preliminary ratings for Army PEBs by VA's Seattle rating site, efforts by the Army to increase MEB staffing, development of Army-wide IDES standardization guidance, and Army-VA electronic records interchange. Periodic meetings are also held between senior Navy medical and VA officials to discuss performance issues at Navy military treatment facilities.

VA holds its own biweekly conferences with local staff responsible for VA's portion of the process. These conferences are supplemented by a bi-weekly IDES "dashboard" that tracks performance data for portions of the IDES for which VA is responsible. According to VA officials, in addition to identifying best practices, these conferences focus on sites with performance problems and identify potential corrective actions. For example, officials said a recent conference addressed delays at Fort Benning, Georgia, and discussed how they could be reduced. VA officials noted that examiner staff were reassigned to this site and worked on weekends to address the problems at this site. In addition, senior VA health care officials hold periodic conferences with officials responsible for exams at IDES sites, to monitor performance.

Ensuring sufficient medical exam resources: In our December 2010 report, we noted that VA struggled to provide enough medical examiners (both VA employees and contractors) to meet demand and deliver exam summaries within its 45-day goal. For example, significant deficiencies in examiner staffing (particularly for mental health exams) at Fort Carson contributed to exams for active duty members taking an average of 140 days. To improve exam timeliness, VA hired more examiners and is devoting more resources at those sites where VA clinicians perform IDES exams. In addition, in July 2011, VA awarded a revised compensation and pension (including IDES) contract that provides more flexibility for VA to have contractors perform IDES exams at sites needing additional resources. As a result, VA can use contractors to conduct exams for regional offices beyond the 10 offices for which the contractor normally provides services. Also, VA contracted with 5 companies to provide short-term exam assistance at IDES sites needing it. Further, VA procedures allow reserve component servicemembers in remote locations to receive exams close to their homes. VA exam timeliness has improved and the agency met its 45-day goal for active component members in every month from August 2011 through June

2012. VA officials attributed improved exam timeliness, in part, to additional exam resources provided to IDES sites. (See app. III for additional information on fiscal year 2012 timeliness.)

Ensuring sufficient exam summaries: In our December 2010 report, we noted that some cases were delayed because VA medical exam summaries were not complete and clear enough for use in making rating and fitness decisions and needed to be sent back to examiners for additional work. VA officials told us that they have been reinforcing the importance of training and communication between rating staff and medical examiners as ways to improve exam summary sufficiency. For example, VA identified types of information which, if missing from an exam summary, would cause it to be insufficient, and has been training examiners to include such information. Additionally, VA noted that VTA now has the ability to track cases with insufficient exams by allowing staff to annotate information on exam summaries. However, staff are not required to provide this information and rules and procedures for its use have not been established.

Ensuring sufficient MEB staffing: In our December 2010 report, we noted that some sites had insufficient MEB physicians, leading to delays in completing the MEB phase. At that time, most of the 27 pilot sites were not meeting the 35-day goal, with average times for active component cases as high as 109 days. Meanwhile, DOD did not have sufficient board liaison staff to handle IDES caseloads. The Army is in the midst of a major hiring initiative intended to more than double staffing for its MEBs over its October 2011 level, which will include additional board liaison and MEB physician positions.[21] The Army reported having 610 full-time equivalent MEB staff positions in October 2011, and planned to hire up to 1,410; this would include 172 MEB physician and 513 board liaison positions. The Army also planned to hire an average of one contact representative per board liaison; these staff members assist the board liaisons with clerical functions, freeing more of the liaisons' time for counseling servicemembers. As of June 2012, the Army had filled 1,219 (86 percent) of the planned 1,410 positions.

Ensuring sufficient VA rating staff: In our December 2010 report, we noted that VA had insufficient staff at one of its rating sites to handle the demand for preliminary ratings, rating reconsiderations, and final VA benefit decisions. VA officials said that the agency has more than tripled the staffing at its IDES rating sites–from 78 to 262 positions. Further, VA has moved staff resources to IDES rating sites from other VA regional offices to provide short-term help in working down rating backlogs. Recent monthly data show an increase in the number of preliminary VA ratings completed, and a slight improvement in processing times. However, as noted before, it is too early to tell the extent to which such trends will continue. (See app. III for additional information on fiscal year 2012 timeliness.)

Improving completeness of reserve component members' records: Service officials noted that incomplete medical records and administrative documentation, especially for reserve component members, often contribute to delays in the early IDES stages, including the VA exam stage. For example, a reserve unit may not have complete medical records for a member who received care from a private provider. When the servicemember enters the IDES, a board liaison is responsible for obtaining the private provider records before handing off the case to VA for exams. To address issues with reserve component servicemembers' records, the Army established an interim office in Pinellas Park, Florida in January 2011. For reserve component servicemembers who may require IDES referral, this office is tasked with obtaining records from the member's reserve unit; reviewing them to identify missing information; and, if necessary, requiring the reserve unit to obtain additional records to complete the case file. Staff at this office also determine whether the member needs IDES referral.[22] Army officials indicated that this office is expected to help reduce the backlog of Army reserve component cases in the IDES. However, Army officials noted that they are providing training to reserve units to improve their ability to maintain complete records on their servicemembers and eventually, the Army may discontinue this office if no longer needed.

Improving MEB documentation and decisions: In response to delays in completing the MEB stage, the Navy and Army have initiatives underway to help ensure the timely completion of narrative summaries and MEB decisions. For example, the Navy piloted electronic narrative summary preparation at Naval Hospital Camp Lejeune, North Carolina. In May 2012, after determining that the piloted process led to improved MEB completion timeliness, the Navy deployed electronic narrative summary preparation Navy-wide. In March 2011, the Army also deployed an abbreviated MEB narrative summary format, intended to provide better information for MEB and PEB decision making while helping reduce delays in the completion of these summaries by MEB clinicians. Incorporating feedback from its MEBs and PEBs, the Army expects the revised IDES template to reduce redundant information, make summaries simpler and easier to use, and standardize summary preparation across their sites.

Resolving diagnostic differences: In our December 2010 report, we identified differences in diagnoses between DOD physicians and VA examiners, especially regarding mental health conditions, as a potential source of delay in IDES. We also noted inconsistencies among services in providing guidance and a lack of a tracking mechanism for determining the extent of diagnostic differences. In response to our recommendation, DOD commissioned a study on the subject. The resulting report confirmed the lack of data on the extent and nature of such differences, and noted that the Army has established guidance more comprehensive than the guidance DOD was developing. It also recommended that DOD or the other services develop similar guidance. A DOD official told us that consistent guidance across the services, similar to the Army's, was included in DOD's December 2011 IDES manual. Also, in response to our recommendation, VA took steps to modify the VTA database used to track IDES to collect information on diagnostic differences. The VTA upgrade was completed in June 2012 after several delays. The report also recommended that DOD and VA establish a committee to improve the accuracy of posttraumatic stress disorder ratings. DOD noted that training on diagnostic differences has been incorporated into its continuing medical education curriculum for military clinicians, but DOD considers the issue of posttraumatic stress disorder ratings largely resolved. Meanwhile, the Army's new IDES narrative summary template includes a section where the MEB clinician identifies any inconsistencies in the case record, including any diagnostic differences with VA examiners.

DOD and VA Are Addressing Shortcomings in Information Systems, but Efforts to Date Are Limited

DOD and VA are working to remedy shortcomings in information systems that support the IDES process. These shortcomings include VTA's lack of capability for local sites to track cases, and the potential for erroneous and missing data in VTA, affecting timeliness measurement. However, some efforts related to information systems are causing work inefficiencies, are still in progress, or otherwise are limited.

Improving local IDES reporting capability: DOD and VA are implementing solutions to improve the ability of local military treatment facilities to track their IDES cases, but multiple initiatives may result in redundant work efforts. Officials told us that the VTA—which is the primary means of tracking the completion of IDES cases—has limited reporting capabilities and staff at local facilities are unable to use it for monitoring the cases for which they are responsible. DOD and VA developed VTA improvements that will allow DOD board liaisons and VA case managers—and their supervisors—to track the status of their cases. VA included these operational reporting improvements in its June 2012 VTA upgrade. In the meantime, staff at many IDES sites have been using their own local systems to track cases and alleviate limitations in VTA. Further, the military services have been moving ahead with their own solutions. For instance, the Army has deployed its own information system for MEBs and PEBs Army-wide. In addition, DOD has also been piloting its own tracking system at 9 IDES sites.[23] As a result, staff at IDES sites we visited reported having to enter the same data into multiple systems. For example, board liaisons at Army MEBs Fort Meade and Joint Base LewisMcChord reported entering data into VTA and the Army's new system, while board liaisons at Andrews Air Force Base reported entering data into VTA and DOD's pilot data system.

Improving IDES data quality: DOD is taking steps to improve the quality of data in VTA. Our analysis of VTA data identified erroneous or missing dates in at least 4 percent of the cases reviewed. Officials told us that VTA lacks adequate controls to prevent erroneous data entry, and that incorrect dates may be entered, or dates may not be entered at all, which can result in inaccurate timeliness data. For example, Army officials noted that some cases shown in VTA as very old were actually closed, but were missing key dates. In September 2011, DOD began a focused effort with the services to correct erroneous and missing case data in VTA. Officials noted that the Air Force and Navy completed substantial efforts to correct the issues identified at that time, but Army efforts continue. DOD and Army officials noted that additional staff resources are being devoted to cleaning up Army VTA data. While improved local tracking and reporting capabilities will help facilities identify and correct erroneous data, keeping VTA data accurate will be an ongoing challenge due to a lack of data entry controls. While DOD is currently assisting the services, DOD officials said they expect that eventually the services will be responsible for identifying and fixing data errors.

DOD and VA are also pursuing options to allow them to save time by replacing the shipping of paper case files among facilities with electronic file transfers. Requirements for an electronic case file transfer solution have been completed and DOD and VA officials expect to begin piloting it in August 2012.

As a short-term solution, the Army and VA began using an Army file transfer Web site to move IDES records between the Army's PEBs and the Seattle VA rating site in March 2012.24 According to VA officials, this could save several days currently spent shipping paper files between these offices. VA officials noted that the same Web site is being used for transfers between the Navy PEB and Providence rating site. Meanwhile, the secretaries of Defense and Veterans Affairs tasked their staffs to develop standards for electronic IDES case files by July 2012.

DOD and VA are Pursuing Broader Solutions to Improving IDES Performance

Based on concerns of the Secretaries of DOD and VA about IDES delays, the departments have undertaken additional initiatives to achieve time savings for servicemembers. For example, in response to the secretaries' February 2011 directive to streamline the process, DOD and VA officials proposed a remodeled IDES process. In December 2011, senior agency leadership decided to postpone the pilot of a remodeled IDES process, and instead tasked the agencies to explore other ways to streamline the process.[25] As a result, DOD, with VA's assistance, began a business process review to better understand how IDES is operating and identify best practices for possible implementation. This review incorporates several efforts, including visits to 8 IDES sites to examine how the process was operating and identify best practices.[26] This review also includes the following:

- *Process simulation model*: Using data from site visits and VTA, DOD is developing a simulation model of the IDES process. According to a DOD official, this process model will allow the agencies to assess the impact of potential situations or changes on IDES processing times, such as surges in workloads or changes in staffing.
- *Fusion diagram*: DOD is developing this diagram to identify the various sources of IDES data—including VA claim forms and narrative summaries—and different information technology systems that play a role in supporting the IDES process. Officials said this diagram would allow them to better understand and identify overlaps and gaps in data systems.

Ultimately, according to DOD officials, this business process review could lead to short- and long-term recommendations to improve IDES performance, potentially including changes to the different steps in the IDES process, performance goals, and staffing levels; and possibly the procurement of a new information system to support process improvements. However, a DOD official noted that these efforts are in their early stages, and thus there is no timetable yet for completing the review or providing recommendations to senior DOD and VA leadership. DOD officials indicated that they expect this to be a continuous IDES improvement process, including further site visits.

Finally, DOD is also developing guidance to expand implementation of an expedited disability evaluation process for servicemembers with catastrophic, combat-related conditions by allowing it to be operated at more military treatment facilities. DOD created this expedited process in January 2009 for servicemembers who suffer catastrophic, combat-related disabilities. Under an agreement with VA, the services can rate such members as 100 percent disabled without the need to use VA's rating schedule. However, according to DOD officials, the services report that no eligible servicemembers are using this process. Instead, servicemembers are having their cases expedited through the IDES informally. The revisions to DOD's policy would allow the expedited process to be used at additional military treatment facilities beyond the original 4 facilities.[27] According to DOD officials, this guidance will be part of a rewrite of DOD's key guidance documents, and was undergoing review at the time of our review.

CONCLUSION

By merging two duplicative disability evaluation systems, IDES shows promise for expediting the delivery of DOD and VA benefits to injured servicemembers and is considered by many to be an improvement over the legacy process it replaced. However, nearly 5 years after its inception as a pilot, delays continue to affect the system and the contribution of various, complex factors to timeliness is not fully understood. Recent efforts by DOD and VA to better understand how different IDES processes contribute to timeliness are promising and may provide the departments with an opportunity to reassess resource levels and timeframes, and to make adjustments if needed. This information will also help to ensure that DOD and VA are making the best use of limited resources to improve IDES performance. However, it is not clear when these efforts will be complete or if any recommended actions will be implemented. DOD has also begun rethinking its approach to determining servicemember satisfaction with IDES. Our analysis of customer satisfaction data suggests that there are opportunities for improving the representativeness of the survey information collected and reconsidering the cost-effectiveness of the current lengthy surveys. Finally, providing local facilities the capability to track and generate reports on the status of their cases is long overdue and may empower local staff to better address challenges. However, tracking reports are only as good as the data that are entered into VTA, and DOD and VA can ensure the quality of these data through continuous monitoring. Meanwhile, the DOD-led business process review should identify and ultimately eliminate any redundant or inefficient information systems for tracking cases as well as for other IDES purposes.

Recommendations for Executive Action

1) To ensure that servicemember cases are processed and are awarded benefits in a timely manner, we recommend that the Secretaries of Defense and Veterans Affairs work together to develop timeframes for completing the IDES business process review and implementing any resulting recommendations.
2) To improve DOD's ability to measure servicemembers' satisfaction with the IDES process, we recommend that the Secretary of Defense develop alternative approaches for collecting more meaningful and representative information in a cost effective manner.
3) To ensure that IDES management decisions continue to be based upon reliable and accurate data, we recommend that the Secretaries of Defense and Veterans Affairs work together to develop a strategy to continuously monitor and remedy issues with VTA timeliness information. This could include issuing guidance to facilities or developing best practices on preventing and correcting data entry errors; and developing reporting capabilities in VTA to alert facilities to potential issues with their data.

Agency Comments and Our Evaluation

We provided a draft of this report to DOD and VA for review and comment. In their written comments, DOD and VA both concurred with our recommendations. VA also provided technical comments, which we incorporated as appropriate. While concurring with our recommendations, DOD also commented that our discussion of IDES surveys contained inaccuracies, but did not specify the inaccurate information in our draft report. In a subsequent communication, DOD officials noted that our draft inaccurately described DOD's decision to not survey veterans. We corrected this information accordingly. Further, while VA concurred with our recommendation that it work with DOD to develop timeframes for completing the IDES business process review and implementing any resulting recommendations, VA stated that DOD is leading the business process review, and therefore should develop the timeframes for completing the review. We have revised this report to clarify that DOD is leading the business process review, but we did not alter the recommendation because we believe that it is important for VA to work closely with DOD, including in developing review timeframes.

Daniel Bertoni
Director,
Education, Workforce, and Income Security Issues

Appendix I: Objectives, Scope, and Methodology

In conducting our review of the Integrated Disability Evaluation System (IDES), our objectives were to examine (1) the extent to which the Departments of Defense (DOD) and Veterans Affairs (VA) are meeting IDES performance goals, and (2) steps DOD and VA are taking to improve IDES performance. We conducted this performance audit from May 2011 to August 2012, in accordance with generally accepted government auditing standards. These standards require that we plan and perform the audit to obtain sufficient, appropriate evidence to provide a reasonable basis for our findings and conclusions based on our audit objectives. We believe the evidence obtained provides a reasonable basis for our findings and conclusions based on our audit objectives.

Review of IDES Timeliness Data

To determine the extent to which IDES is meeting established timeliness goals, we analyzed data collected through VA's Veterans Tracking Application (VTA) database. While VA manages VTA, both DOD and VA staff enter data into VTA, and the evaluation of IDES data is primarily conducted by staff at DOD's Office of Warrior Care Policy (WCP).1 WCP provided us with a dataset that was current as of January 1, 2012 and contained data spanning back to the inception of IDES in late 2007. This data export included data on a total of 39,260 cases. Of these cases, 34,185 were active duty servicemembers and 5,068 were Reserve/Guard servicemembers.2 This VTA data set contained demographic data for each individual IDES case as well as a record of dates for when servicemembers reached various milestones in IDES.3 Overall and interim IDES timeliness calculations are based on computing the number of days elapsed between appropriate milestone dates. For example, overall timeliness for servicemembers that receive benefits is calculated as the number of days between the individual being referred into the IDES and the date on which his or her VA benefits letter is issued. We met with staff at WCP to ensure we used appropriate variables when calculating timeliness. We also met with officials at VA to discuss the calculations used to determine the timeliness of cases.

We took a number of steps to assess the reliability of VTA data and ultimately found the data to be sufficiently reliable for the purposes of our audit. Past GAO work[4] relied on VTA data, and therefore we took a number of steps to follow up on past assessments of VTA.

- We interviewed DOD and VA and determined that internal controls on VTA data had not changed substantially since our past review.
- We conducted electronic testing of the VTA data and generally found low rates of missing data or erroneous dates pertinent to our analysis—approximately 4 percent of cases. [5] For IDES cases in which we found missing dates or dates out of sequence, we excluded those cases from all of our analyses. While there were some instances in which the erroneous dates may be justified, we excluded the entire case from our analysis if any such dates appeared at any point in the VTA database. Such data included cases in which (1) there was no MEB referral date signifying the start of IDES process, and (2) the ending date preceded the beginning date of the IDES phase (resulting in timeliness calculations appearing as a negative amount of time).
- We also conducted a limited trace-to-file process to determine whether date fields in VTA were an accurate reflection of the information in IDES case files. Specifically, we compared VTA dates in 15 IDES cases completed in fiscal year 2011 against the dates in the corresponding paper files. In comparing dates, we allowed for a discrepancy of 5 days in dates to allow for the possibility that dates

may have been entered into the database after an event took place. Ninety-three percent of the dates we traced back to the original file documents were found to be accurate, that is falling within our 5 day allowance.

Analysis Conducted Using VTA Data

For the cases meeting our criteria for reliability, we analyzed timeliness data for those cases that had completed the entire IDES process or had completed each of the four IDES phases. We specifically:

- Identified the total number of cases enrolled each fiscal year[6] from FY 2008 through 2011, by active as well as National Guard and reserve servicemembers, and by military branch of service.[7]
- Identified the number of cases that completed the entire IDES process for each fiscal year from fiscal year 2008 through fiscal year 2011. We analyzed completed cases in two different ways: (1) those who completed the process and received VA benefits and (2) those who completed the IDES with any outcome (such as permanent retirement, Temporary Disability Retirement List, return to duty, etc.). In order to be able to make comparisons across cases with different outcomes for a given point in time, we defined fiscal year by using the VTA variable "final disposition date". We did this because most completed cases—regardless of outcome—have a final disposition date in VTA. In contrast to our approach, VA use the "VA benefit date" variable to determine fiscal year of completion for cases resulting in benefits. As such, their number of cases and timeliness calculations by fiscal year differed from ours, although overall trends are similar.
- Identified the number of cases that completed each phase of IDES and the interim stages within each phase, again by fiscal year (fiscal years 2008 through 2011).
- Computed timeliness statistics for the completion of the IDES process, phases, and stages against the performance goals set by DOD and VA, such as average days and percent meeting goals.
- Computed number and percent of cases where a servicemember appealed a decision made during the IDES process, by fiscal year.

For the purposes of this report, GAO opted to not include reserve component time spent in the VA benefit phase in our calculations for overall time because the 30 days allotted for this phase is not included in the 305-day overall goal for the reserve component.

GAO also performed analyses similar to those above, except that we grouped cases according to the year in which they were enrolled in IDES. (See app. II for more detail on these analyses.) Additionally, we analyzed timeliness for cases that had not yet completed the MEB stage as of the date we received the VTA data.

Review of IDES Customer Satisfaction Data

To determine the extent to which IDES is meeting its customer satisfaction goals, we analyzed data collected from IDES customer satisfaction surveys conducted at the end of three phases: MEB, PEB and Transition. These surveys are administered by telephone by contractors hired by DOD. The dataset we received contained survey responses for individual servicemembers from the beginning of the IDES pilot to December 2011, at which time administration of the survey was suspended. Additionally, we matched individual survey responses with information from VTA to gain additional understanding into how customer satisfaction varied according to different factors such as timeliness and case outcome. We matched survey and VTA data using the unique case identifier attached to each IDES case, maintaining the anonymity of the servicemembers. See appendix II for the results of additional analyses we conducted using survey data and survey data matched with VTA data.

In the course of our review we concluded that the survey data were sufficiently reliable for our purposes. We interviewed relevant officials at DOD and their contractors about eligibility requirements and the administration of the surveys. Further, we met with DOD and their contractors on multiple occasions to discuss the calculations used to determine response rates for the survey and servicemembers' level of satisfaction. See appendix II for more details on GAO's review of response rates.

Identifying Challenges and Actions Taken to Improve Performance

To identify challenges in implementing IDES as well as steps taken to improve performance, we visited six military treatment facilities. During the site visits, we interviewed officials involved in implementing IDES from both DOD and VA, including military facility commanders and administrators, DOD board liaisons, military physicians involved in MEB determinations, DOD legal staff, VA case workers, VA or contract examiners, and administrators at VA medical clinics and regional offices. Additionally, we interviewed servicemembers who were currently enrolled in the IDES process. We selected the six facilities to obtain perspectives from sites in different military services, geographic areas, and their ability to meet timeliness goals for different phases of the process (see table 7). In addition, we visited the Air Force's Formal Physical Evaluation Board at Randolph Air Force Base, Texas. During this visit we observed a hearing and met with board members to obtain a better understanding of the process.

Table 7. Selected Characteristics of IDES Pilot Sites Visited as of May 2011

Military treatment facility	Military service	State	IDES caseload	Average exam times (goal = 45 days)	Average MEB stage times (goal = 35 days)	Average Total IDES time (goal = 295 days)
Joint Base Andrews	Air Force	Maryland	511	24	56	472
Fort Hood	Army	Texas	1,976	31	107	334
Joint Base Lewis-McChord	Army	Washington	1,069	46	102	339
Fort Meade	Army	Maryland	543	35	140	556
Fort Sam Houston	Army	Texas	1,336	65	72	412
Naval Hospital Bremerton	Navy	Washington	199	52	14	348

Source: GAO analysis of DOD's June 2011 IDES Monthly Report.
Note: Processing times listed in table are for active duty cases.

We also interviewed officials in various offices at DOD and VA involved in implementing IDES. At DOD, these offices included Warrior Care Policy; Office of the Assistant Secretary of Defense (Reserve Affairs); Office of the Deputy Chief Management Officer; Air Force Physical Disability Division; Army Physical Disability Agency; Navy Physical Evaluation Board; Air Force Surgeon General; Army Medical Command; and Navy Bureau of Medicine and Surgery. At VA, we interviewed officials in the Veterans Benefits

Administration, Veterans Health Administration, and the VA/DOD Collaboration Service. Furthermore, we reviewed relevant documents, including DOD and VA policies, federal laws, regulations, directives[8] and guidance, a study produced for DOD on diagnostic variances, and plans to streamline IDES or improve performance.

APPENDIX II: ADDITIONAL TIMELINESS AND SATISFACTION ANALYSES

This appendix provides additional information on the timeliness of the IDES process and servicemember satisfaction with it. First, we use timeliness data to examine whether changes over time in processing times and the percentage of cases meeting timeliness goals look any different when cases are grouped according to the fiscal year in which the cases were first enrolled rather than the fiscal year in which the cases were completed.[1]

Second, we use survey data to examine different measurements of servicemember satisfaction with IDES, how satisfaction varied according to various servicemember characteristics, response and coverage rates for the servicemembers surveyed, and how the survey respondents differed from nonrespondents.[2]

With respect to timeliness, we find generally similar trends for cases grouped by fiscal year of enrollment versus fiscal year of completion, with some key differences.

Organizing cases by completion date results in shorter average processing times in 2008, since only those cases that are processed quickly could be completed in the first year of IDES. As such, organizing cases by enrollment date provides a better estimate of the processing times for the early IDES cases. However, this approach results in shorter processing times in 2011, the most recent full year of the program, since only cases that finish quickly can be analyzed.

With respect to satisfaction, we find that the particular index used to summarize servicemembers' responses can affect the proportion reported as being "satisfied" or "dissatisfied" with IDES overall. DOD's index suggests that 67 percent of servicemembers have been satisfied since the IDES program began, but a reasonable alternative measure we developed suggests that only 24 percent of servicemembers have been satisfied. Using this measure, satisfaction varies only slightly across many important groups of servicemembers, such as by disenrollment outcome, suggesting that available program data cannot precisely explain satisfaction outcomes. Also, servicemembers surveyed may not represent the servicemembers who completed the different phases of IDES well enough to generalize to them, given the low response rates to the MEB survey and fact that being selected for latter (PEB and Transition) surveys were conditional on completing the MEB survey.

Overall IDES Timeliness: Processing Times and Percent of Cases Meeting Timeliness Goals

Average IDES processing times for completed cases resulting in benefits generally worsened since 2008, especially for active duty cases, regardless of whether cases are grouped by the fiscal year in which they were completed (fig. 10) or by the fiscal year in which they were enrolled (fig. 11). The notable exception is when fiscal year 2011 is the year of enrollment. However, caution must be used when examining cases enrolled in 2011 because over 15,600 service members of the 18,651 (or at least 84 percent) who entered IDES in fiscal year 2011 did not have an outcome in 2011 and were enrolled in IDES as of January 1, 2012,[3] potentially changing the distribution of processing times as they proceed through IDES.

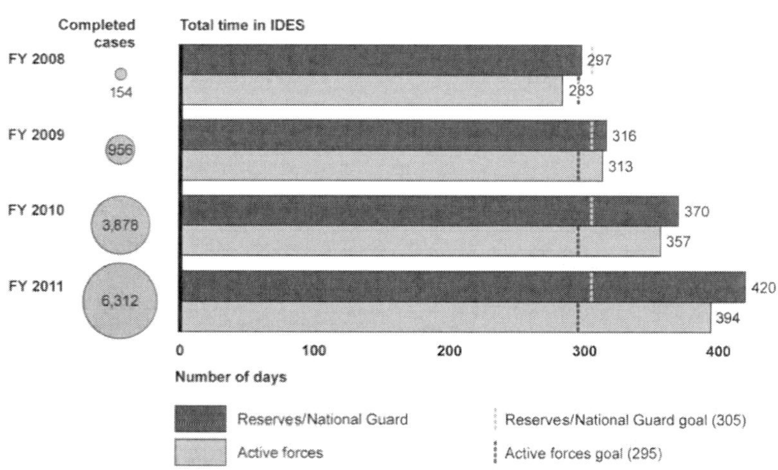

Source: GAO analysis of DOD and VA data.

Figure 10. Average IDES Processing Times by Year of Completion, for Completed Cases Resulting in Benefits.

We also examine average IDES processing times according to year of completion (see figure 12) and year of enrollment for cases (see figure 13) for all completed cases regardless of outcome. As with cases that resulted in benefits, for cases resulting in any outcome we find that average processing times increased since 2008—again with the exception of fiscal year 2011 for reasons discussed earlier—although average processing times are somewhat shorter than when only servicemembers receiving benefits are included (figure 11).

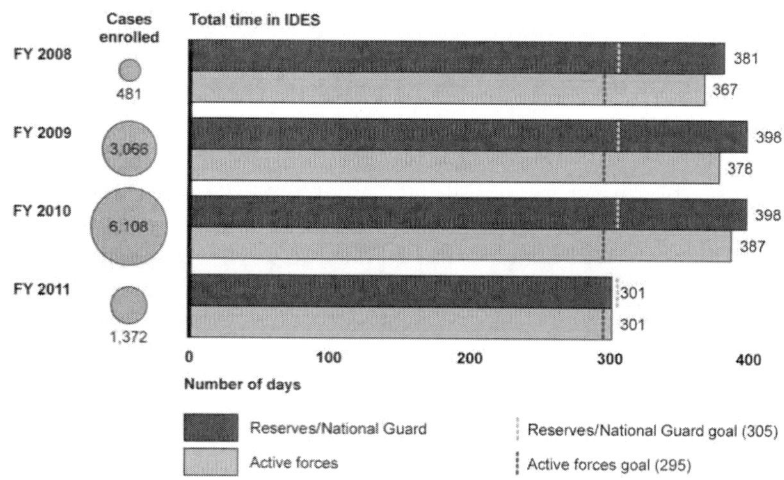

Source: GAO analysis of DOD and VA data.

Note: Enrolled cases reflects those cases that were enrolled for each year with cases with erroneous or questionable dates removed. This number does not match the number of enrolled cases previously reported for this reason.

Figure 11. Average IDES Processing Times by Fiscal Year of Enrollment for Completed Cases Resulting in Benefits.

Figures 14 and 15 show that regardless of whether cases are organized by year of completion or enrollment, the percent of completed cases resulting in benefits that were not timely increased between fiscal year 2008 and 2010 for both active duty servicemembers and members in the Reserves or National Guard. As with the average processing times, caution must be used when examining cases enrolled in fiscal year 2011 (fig. 15), since only those cases that are processed quickly are observed in the last year. Similarly, caution also must be used when examining cases in 2008 (fig. 14), since the only cases that are included in the first year are those that completed IDES quickly.

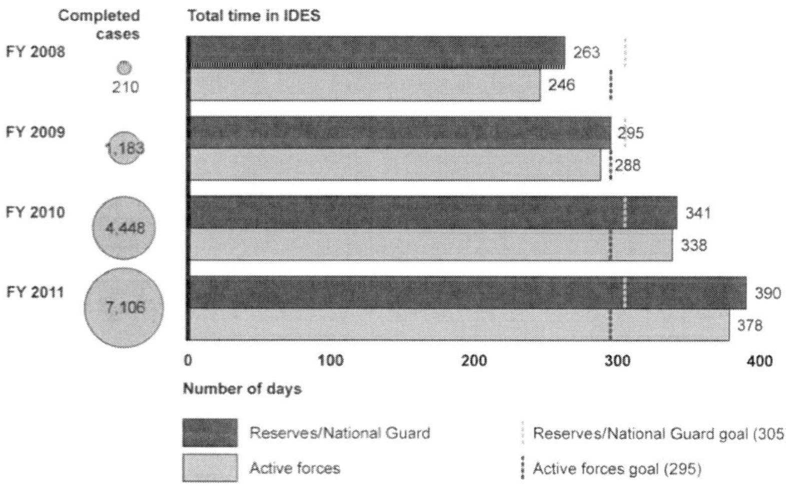

Source: GAO analysis of DOD and VA data.

Figure 12. Average IDES Processing Times by Year of Completion, for All Completed Cases Regardless of Outcome.

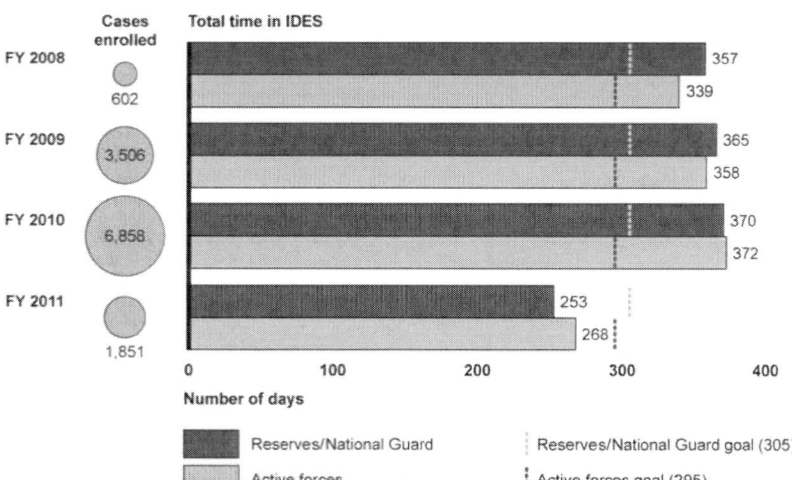

Source: GAO analysis of DOD and VA data.

Note: Enrolled cases reflects those cases that were enrolled for each year with cases with erroneous or questionable dates removed. This number does not match the number of enrolled cases previously reported for this reason.

Figure 13. Average IDES Processing Times by Fiscal Year of Enrollment for All Completed Cases Regardless of Outcome.

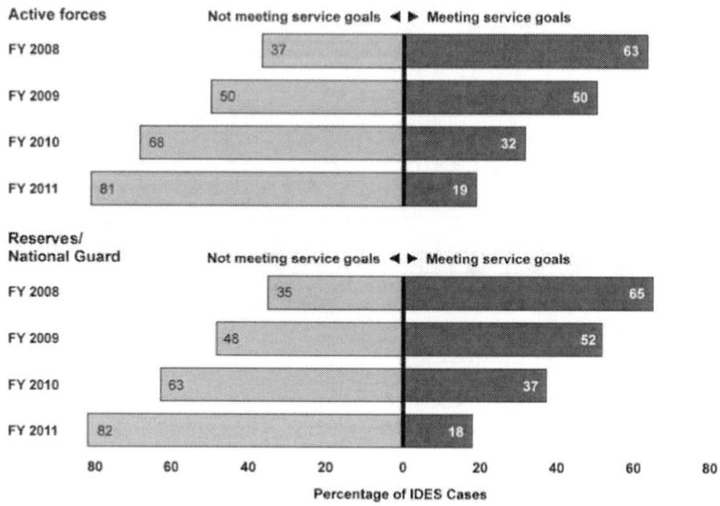

Source: GAO analysis of DOD and VA data.

Figure 14. Percentage of Completed Cases Meeting and Missing the Overall Processing Time Goals, by Fiscal Year of IDES Completion, for Servicemembers Receiving Benefits.

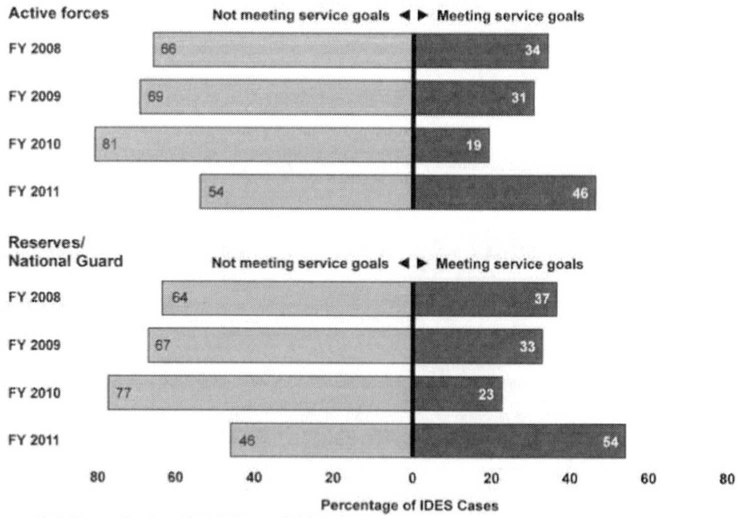

Source: GAO analysis of DOD and VA data.

Figure 15. Percentage of Completed Cases Meeting and Missing the Overall Processing Time Goals, by Fiscal Year of IDES Enrollment, for Servicemembers Receiving Benefits.

Figures 16 and 17 show how average processing times for each of the four phases of IDES have changed over the four fiscal years when cases are grouped by the fiscal year in which they completed a given phase and when cases are grouped by the fiscal year in which they were enrolled or started a given phase.[4] Figure 16 shows that when cases are grouped according to the fiscal year in which the different phases were completed, processing times increased for all phases except the Transition phase.

Figure 17 shows a roughly similar pattern of increases in processing times in all but the Transition phase, though processing times in 2011 are skewed for the reason mentioned above.

Figures 18 and 19 show how the percentages meeting the timeliness goals for each of the four phases of IDES have changed over the four fiscal years when cases are grouped by the fiscal year in which they completed a given phase and when cases are grouped by the fiscal year in which they were enrolled or started a given phase.

Figure 18 shows that the percent of cases meeting timeliness goals decreased over the four years for the MEB and PEB phases, although a high percent of cases met PEB goals. However, the Transition and Benefits phases fluctuated up and down and both were favorable across some years. Figure 19 also shows decreases in percentages of cases meeting timeliness goals at the MEB and PEB phases when cases are grouped by fiscal year of starting a given phase. The fluctuations in the timeliness of the Transition and Benefits phases were more prevalent when cases were grouped in this manner.

Servicemember Satisfaction Survey: Response and Coverage Rates

Low response and coverage rates for servicemember satisfaction surveys administered after each phase of IDES raise concerns about how well the satisfaction survey results represented the larger population of servicemembers who completed one or more phases.

DOD surveys servicemembers after they complete the MEB, PEB, and Transition phases of IDES. The department attempts to survey all servicemembers who complete each phase, but only if they completed the prior surveys. For example, the MEB survey must be completed before a servicemember is eligible to complete the PEB survey.

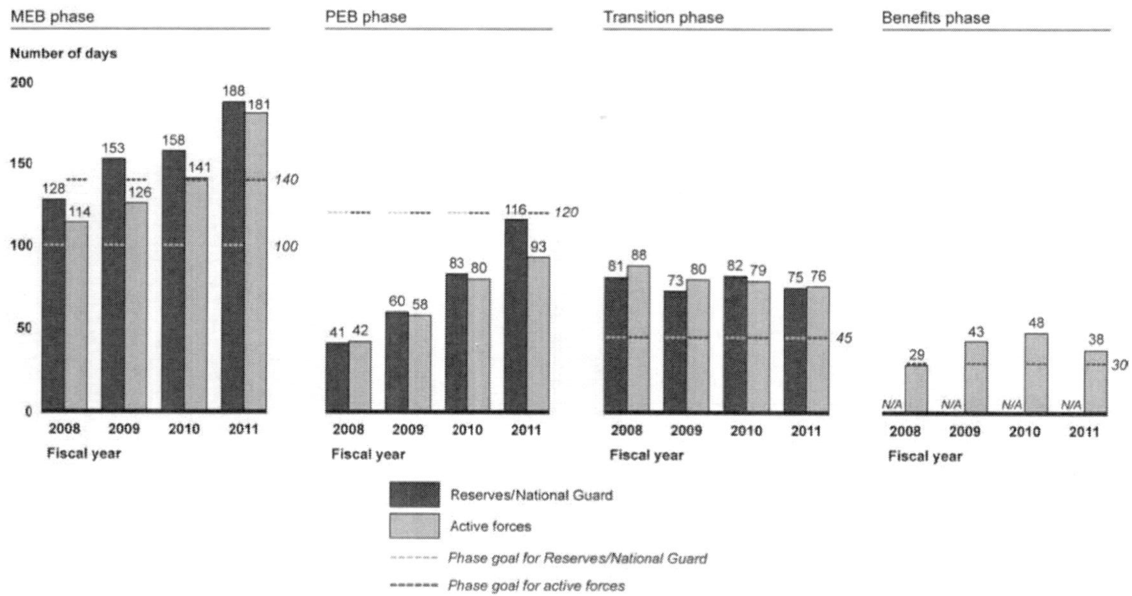

Source: GAO analysis of DOD and VA data.

Note: Data shown in figures 16, 17, 18, and 19 are for servicemember cases that either started or completed a phase in a particular year, according to the figure title. For purposes of this report, we opted to not include reserve component time spent in the VA benefit phase in our calculations phase because this goal applies to some but not all reservists, depending on their active duty status. Any time spent within the VA benefit phase is reflected within the overall processing time calculations for such reserve component servicemembers.

Figure 16. Average Processing Time for Each IDES Phase, by Fiscal Year in Which the Phase Was Completed.

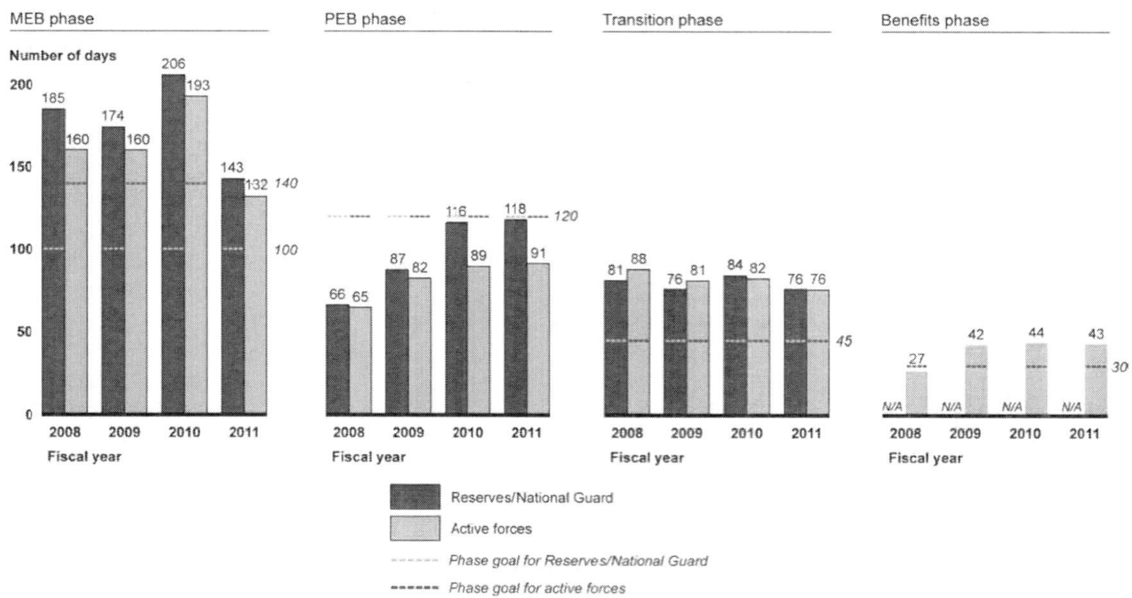

Source: GAO analysis of DOD and VA data.

Note: Data shown in figures 16, 17, 18, and 19 are for servicemember cases that either started or completed a phase in a particular year, according to the figure title. For purposes of this report, we opted to not include reserve component time spent in the VA benefit phase in our calculations phase because this goal applies to some but not all reservists, depending on their active duty status. Any time spent within the VA benefit phase is reflected within the overall processing time calculations for such reserve component servicemembers.

Figure 17. Average Processing Time for Each IDES Phase, by Fiscal Year of Enrollment in Each Phase.

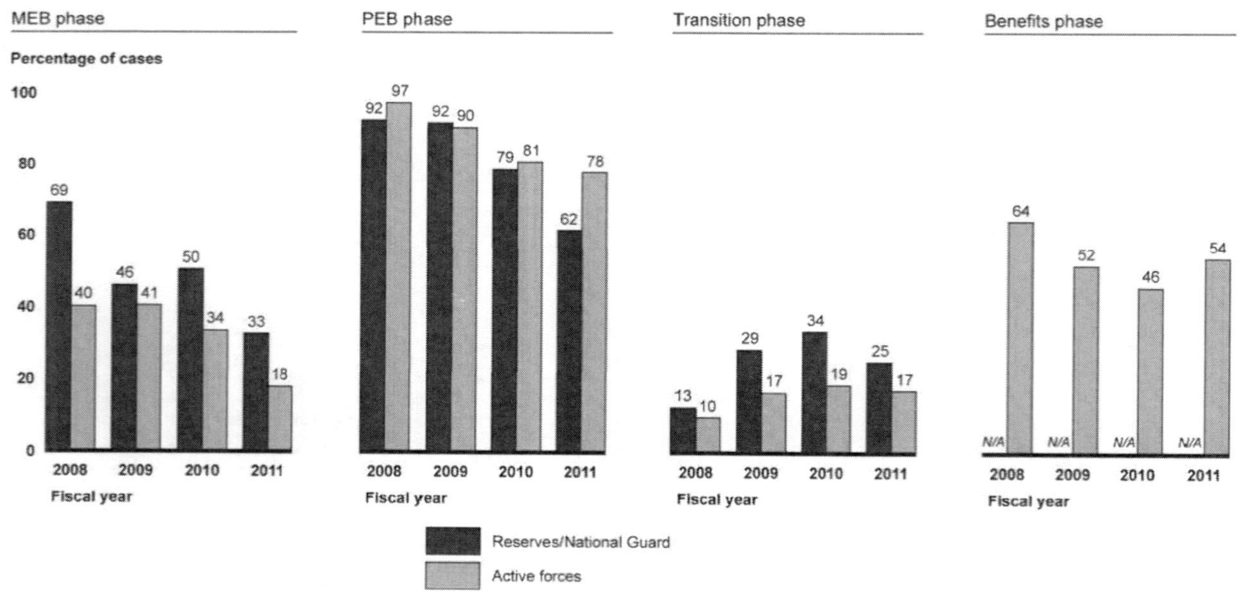

Source: GAO analysis of DOD and VA data.

Note: Data shown in figures 16, 17, 18, and 19 are for servicemember cases that either started or completed a phase in a particular year, according to the figure title. For purposes of this report, we opted to not include reserve component time spent in the VA benefit phase in our calculations phase because this goal applies to some but not all reservists, depending on their active duty status. Any time spent within the VA benefit phase is reflected within the overall processing time calculations for such reserve component servicemembers.

Figure 18. Percent of Cases Meeting Timeliness Goals for each Phase of IDES, by Fiscal Year in Which the Phase Was Completed.

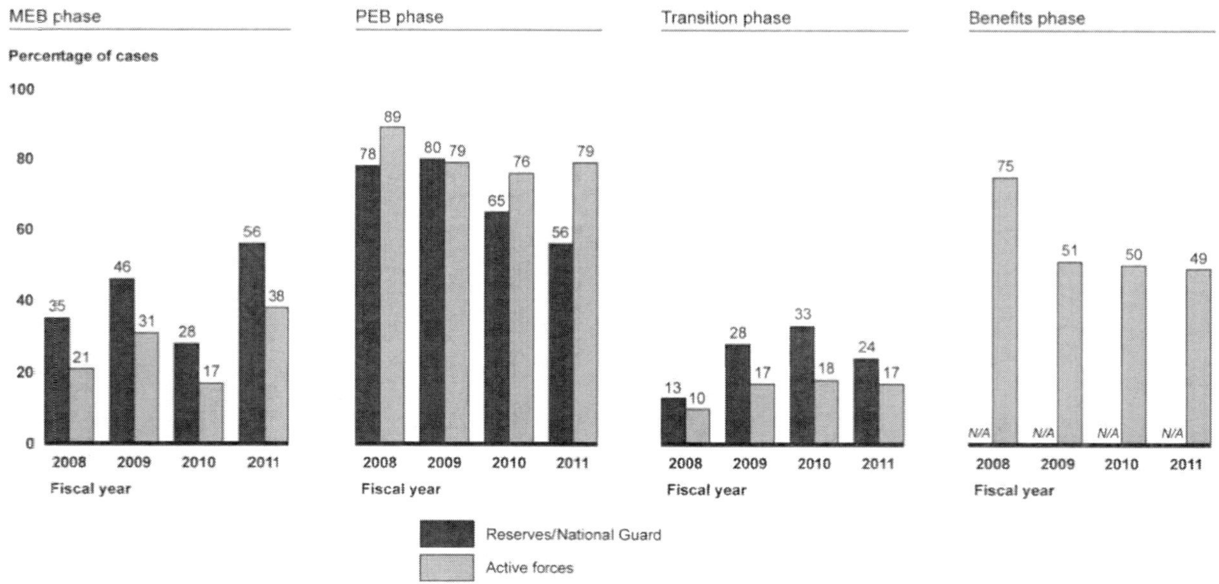

Source: GAO analysis of DOD and VA data.

Note: Data shown in figures 16, 17, 18, and 19 are for servicemember cases that either started or completed a phase in a particular year, according to the figure title. For purposes of this report, we opted to not include reserve component time spent in the VA benefit phase in our calculations phase because this goal applies to some but not all reservists, depending on their active duty status. Any time spent within the VA benefit phase is reflected within the overall processing time calculations for such reserve component servicemembers.

Figure 19. Percent of Cases Meeting Timeliness Goals for each Phase of IDES, by Fiscal Year of Enrollment in Each Phase.

Using the data available to us, and as table 8 below shows, we found that 9,604 of the 25,212 servicemembers who completed the MEB phase were surveyed, for a 38 percent response and coverage rate.5 Of the 18,296 servicemembers who completed the PEB phase, only 8,968 of them completed the prior MEB survey and were eligible for the PEB survey and of these only 4,795 were surveyed. Using DOD's eligibility criteria, the response rate for the PEB survey was roughly 54 percent (4,795 of 8,968).

However, the coverage rate for all servicemembers who completed the PEB phase (regardless of whether they completed the prior survey) was only 26 percent (4,795 of 18,296). Similarly, the response rate for the Transition survey was 72 percent while the coverage rate was only 23 percent (See table 8).

Table 8. Survey phase response and coverage rates

Phase	Service members completing phase	Service members eligible for survey (completed prior phase survey)	Service members surveyed	Response rate (No. surveyed / No. eligible) (%)	Coverage rate(No. surveyed / No.completin g phase) (%)
MEB	25,212	all	9,604	38.1%	38.1%
PEB	18,296	8,968	4,795	53.5%	26.2%
Transition	12,352	3,996	2,893	72.4%	23.4%

Source: GAO analysis of DOD and VA data.

Note: This table excludes 558 cases (or approximately 1.4 percent) of VTA data with logical errors in IDES phase start and end days for any IDES phase (e.g. exclude cases where MEB start date occurs after MEB end date). This table includes the approximately 4 percent of cases we found to have inconsistent start and end dates across phases.

As table 9 below shows, there were some sizable differences between respondents and nonrespondents, especially for the PEB and Transition surveys. For example, respondents to the transition survey spent more time than nonrespondents in the Transition phase, were less likely to be separated with benefits, and were more likely to be placed on the Permanent Disability Retired List.

These differences, combined with low response and coverage rates, raise the possibility of biased responses.

Table 9. Selected Servicemember Characteristics of Respondents and Nonrespondents to the MEB, PEB and Transition Surveys

Survey	Variable	Respondents		Nonrespondents	
		N	Mean or percent	N	Mean or percent
MEB survey	Timeliness				
	Total days in MEB	9,604	158.8	15,608	156.6
	Met MEB goal	2,854	29.7%	5,187	33.2%
	Branch				
	Army	5,191	54.1%	8,910	57.1%
	Marine Corps	2,177	22.7%	2,802	18.0%
	Navy	1,417	14.8%	2,168	13.9%
	US Air Force	819	8.5%	1,728	11.1%
	Component				
	Active duty	8,628	89.8%	14,111	90.4%
	Reserve/National Guard	976	10.2%	1,497	9.6%
	Outcome of case				
	Separated with benefits	2,778	31.4%	2,678	31.0%
	Separated without benefits	152	1.7%	134	1.6%
	Permanent disability retirement list	2,191	24.7%	2,192	25.3%
	Temporary disability retirement list	2,704	30.5%	2,730	31.6%
	Found fit and returned to duty	959	10.8%	856	9.9%
	Found unfit and returned to duty	73	0.8%	61	0.7%
PEB Survey	Timeliness				
	Total days in PEB	4,764	85.0	13,364	91.2
	Met PEB goal	3,762	79.0%	10,424	78.0%
	Branch				
	Army	2,646	55.5%	8,298	62.1%
	Marine Corps	1,061	22.3%	2,347	17.6%
	Navy	708	14.9%	1,640	12.3%
	US Air Force	349	7.3%	1,079	8.1%
	Component				
	Active duty	4,262	89.5%	12,228	91.5%
	Reserve/National Guard	502	10.54	1,136	8.50
	Outcome of case				

Table 9. (Continued)

Survey	Variable	Respondents N	Respondents Mean or percent	Nonrespondents N	Nonrespondents Mean or percent
	Separated with benefits	1,408	29.6%	4,035	31.9%
	Separated without benefits	72	1.51	211	1.7%
	Permanent disability retirement list	1,222	25.7%	3,147	24.9%
	Temporary disability retirement list	1,440	30.2%	3,962	31.4%
	Found fit and returned to duty	584	12.3%	1,181	9.4%
	Found unfit and returned to duty	38	0.8%	94	0.7%
Transition survey	Timeliness				
	Total days in transition	2,894	82.3	9,259	75.1
	Met transition goal	455	15.7%	1,856	20.0%
	Branch				
	Army	1,744	60.3%	5,972	64.5%
	Marine Corps	597	20.6%	1,837	19.8%
	Navy	344	11.9%	924	10.0%
	US Air Force	209	7.2%	526	5.7%
	Component				
	Active Duty	2,587	89.4%	8,562	92.5%
	Reserve/National Guard	307	10.6%	697	7.5%
	Outcome of Case				
	Separated with benefits	783	27.1%	3,496	38.1%
	Separated without benefits	47	1.6%	173	1.9%
	Permanent disability retirement list	955	33.0%	2,405	26.2%
	Temporary disability retirement list	1,102	38.1%	3,086	33.7%
	Found fit and returned to duty	5	0.2%	4	0.0%
	Found unfit and returned to duty	2	0.1%	3	0.0%

Source: GAO analysis of DOD and VA data.

Note: This table excludes 558 cases (or approximately 1.4 percent) of VTA data with logical errors in IDES phase start and end days, for any IDES phase (e.g. exclude cases where MEB start date occurs after MEB end date). This table includes the approximately 4 percent of cases we found to have inconsistent start and end dates across phases.

Measuring Servicemember Satisfaction

The particular measure used to assess servicemember satisfaction can affect the proportion reported as "satisfied" with the IDES program. Depending on the measure used, satisfaction is about 2.8 times lower than what DOD has reported, and many servicemembers classified as "satisfied" express moderate dissatisfaction with some aspects of the process.

DOD has reported average servicemember satisfaction with IDES overall and with three phases of the process, i.e., MEB, PEB, and Transition phases. In so doing, DOD has developed indices of satisfaction on several broad dimensions, such as satisfaction with the overall experience and fairness, which combine responses to selected survey questions. Although the number of questions used in each index vary depending on the number of phases completed, each index classifies servicemembers as "satisfied" or "dissatisfied" using the average of their responses across all questions in the index. Each question's scale ranges from 1 to 5, with 1 denoting "very dissatisfied" (or a similar negative response), 5 denoting "very satisfied," and 3 denoting "neither satisfied nor dissatisfied." DOD reports that a servicemember is "satisfied" if his or her average response across all items in the scale exceeds 3. Table 10 summarizes the responses to each question that DOD uses in its overall satisfaction index at each phase (as of August 2011).

DOD's indices are one reasonable method of summarizing servicemember opinions. In quarterly performance reports, DOD notes that it has used factor analysis, a form of latent variable statistical models to assess the reliability of its scales. While we did not review DOD's models, we independently found that DOD's overall index of satisfaction with IDES was highly reliable. (Specifically, using Cronbach's alpha, the index was highly correlated with a single latent dimension at $\alpha = 0.92$.) This supports DOD's choice to measure the single concept of "satisfaction" by averaging the ordinal servicemember responses.

Nevertheless, the average survey response can obscure variation in the responses that make up the index. For example, suppose that a servicemember said she was "very satisfied" (response of 5) on two of the four questions in the index, "dissatisfied" on one (response of 2) and "very dissatisfied" on the last one (response of 1). With an average response over 3, the DOD measure would classify her as "satisfied," despite the fact that she was "somewhat dissatisfied" or "very dissatisfied" with two of the four aspects of IDES that DOD considers important.

Table 10. Questions Used in DOD Indices of Overall Servicemember Satisfaction

	MEB phase			*PEB phase*				*Transition phase*
	Number	*Percent*		*Number*	*Percent*	*Number*		*Percent*
How satisfied or dissatisfied were you with the management of your case during the [MEB/PEB/Transition] phase of the pilot process?								
Very dissatisfied	813	8.4		388	7.9		223	6.4
Dissatisfied	1,369	14.1		607	12.4		406	11.6
Neither	1,259	13		578	11.8		397	11.3
Satisfied	4,310	44.5		2,306	47.1		1,737	49.6
Very satisfied	1,926	19.9		1,019	20.8		741	21.1
Total	*9,677*	*100*		*4,898*	*100*		*3,504*	*100*
How satisfied or dissatisfied were you with the overall [MEB/PEB/Transition] phase of determining your retention status?								
Very dissatisfied	559	6.7		269	5.5		224	6.4
Dissatisfied	1,131	13.6		548	11.2		401	11.5
Neither	1,007	12.1		510	10.4		345	9.9
Satisfied	4,048	48.6		2,562	52.3		1,798	51.6
Very satisfied	1,578	19		1014	20.7		715	20.5
Total	*8,323*	*100*		*4,903*	*100*		*3,483*	*100*
How would you evaluate the timeliness of the process since entering the Disability Evaluation Pilot process?								
Very poor	1,685	17.4		759	15.4		500	14.1
Poor	1,594	16.5		681	13.9		468	13.2
Mix of poor/good	2,397	24.7		1,262	25.7		967	27.3
Good	2,811	29		1,470	29.9		1,065	30.1
Very good	1,200	12.4		743	15.1		543	15.3
Total	*9,687*	*100*		*4,915*	*100*		*3,543*	*100*
How would you evaluate your overall experience since entering the Disability Evaluation Pilot process?								
Very poor	686	7		356	7.2		235	6.6
Poor	921	9.4		413	8.4		285	8
Mix of poor/good	2,875	29.4		1,477	29.9		1,115	31.4
Good	3,891	39.8		1,917	38.8		1,333	37.5
Very good	1,402	14.3		772	15.6		587	16.5
Total	*9,775*	*100*		*4,935*	*100*		*3,555*	*100*

Source: GAO analysis of DOD data.

Note: Entries are responses to four survey questions (rows) asked after servicemembers complete the MEB, PEB, or Transition phase (columns).

The grouping rule considers this servicemember equally happy with IDES as someone who says they are "satisfied" with all four aspects in the index.

To assess the extent to which DOD's index might mask dissatisfaction, we calculated the proportion of questions in the scale on which servicemembers whom DOD classified as "satisfied" gave neutral or negative responses (1, 2, or 3). We found that half of these servicemembers gave neutral or negative answers to at least 25 percent of the items in the index, and a quarter gave such answers to at least 41 percent of the items. For these servicemembers, the DOD index may suggest more satisfaction than the underlying survey questions would support.

We further assessed the sensitivity of DOD's index by comparing it against a different (i.e., GAO's) measure of satisfaction: whether a servicemember is "somewhat" or "very satisfied" (or gives a similarly positive response) on all items in DOD's scale of overall IDES satisfaction. Our measure is more conservative than DOD's, because ours only includes positive responses and uses a broader cutpoint (two response categories) to distinguish between "satisfied" and "not satisfied" servicemembers. (In contrast, DOD calculates average satisfaction on an ordinal scale of 1 to 5, and then uses a cutpoint at 3.) Our measure is not inherently more valid, however, and has its own weaknesses. In particular, we classify a servicemember as "not satisfied" if she gives a neutral or negative response to just one of the four items in DOD's scale.[6]

When we analyzed overall satisfaction using both measures, we found that overall, servicemembers are 2.8 times less satisfied on our measure than on DOD's (i.e., 23.8 versus 67 percent). Further, only about 20 to 30 percent of servicemembers are "satisfied" with each aspect of the IDES process that DOD considers important across most of the subgroups we analyzed, while DOD classifies about 60 to 70 percent of such servicemembers as "satisfied" on average. In the next section, we present further information on variation in satisfaction across servicemember groups.

Explaining Servicemember Satisfaction Outcomes

Although the servicemember survey provides numerous measures of satisfaction, it is also important to explain variation in satisfaction outcomes i.e. why some servicemembers are more satisfied than others. Explaining variation can connect dissatisfaction with poor program performance and help identify specific reforms to improve the experiences of servicemembers who typically have been less satisfied. However, the available program data cannot precisely explain outcomes when used in this type of explanatory analysis. Using the available data, we could predict satisfaction only 1.9 percentage points better after controlling for multiple factors than what we would have achieved by chance (65.5 percent vs. 63.7 percent of satisfied responses predicted correctly).

In order to further explain variation in satisfaction, we matched the survey responses to the data that DOD and VA maintain on the processing of each servicemember's case, known as the VTA data. This database primarily measures the time it took servicemembers to complete each phase of the IDES process. A small number of other program and demographic variables are also available, such as service branch, component, and the number of conditions claimed and referred. Using the matched survey and VTA data, we estimated the association between satisfaction and observable factors that could potentially explain variation in servicemembers' experiences.

Table 11 below (columns 2-4) presents these associations for both DOD's and GAO's overall measures of satisfaction. The "raw data" estimates are simply the proportion of servicemembers in a particular group who were satisfied according to either measure. In the fourth column ("model estimates"), we estimate this proportion holding constant all of the other factors listed, using a statistical model.

Table 11. Overall IDES Satisfaction by Subgroups

	DOD Measure: Average answer exceeded neutral	GAO Measure: All answers positive		N
	Raw data	Raw data	Model estimates	
	Percentage	Percentage	Percentage	
All respondents	67	23.8		9,865
Component				
Active	67.4	23.7	23.7	8,692
Reserves/National Guard	63.5	24.6	23.7	1,173
Branch				
Air Force	61.8	23.6	23.7	838
Army	70.3	26.5	24.5	5,398
Marine Corps	61.3	19	23.8	2,198
Navy	65.9	21.2	23	1,431

	DOD Measure: Average answer exceeded neutral	GAO Measure: All answers positive		N
	Raw data	Raw data	Model estimates	
	Percentage	Percentage	Percentage	
Rollout phase[a]				
1	63.7	20.2		1,430
1.1	65.1	21.8		4,827
2	72.7	30.4		1,601
3.1	69.6	34.6		257
3.2	67.7	38.5		65
3.3	0	0		1
Final disposition				
Fit and Returned to Duty	70.9	27.4	21.7	963
Permanent Disability	69.9	25.4	25.6	2,286
Separated with Benefits	66.9	23.1	22.5	2,848
Separated without Benefits	63.1	20.4	21.5	157
Temporary Disability	65.9	21.8	24.4	2,786
Unfit and Returned to Duty	63	16.4	17	73
Fiscal Year started MEB				
2008	60.4	15.1	13	530
2009	68.1	21.4	21.2	2,627
2010	66.1	22.9	24.5	4,721
2011	69.3	31.6	28.3	1,986
Claimed conditions				
0-4	71.5	27.7	24.2	2,309
5-7	69.4	25.1	23.9	2,028
8-12	65.9	22.5	23.1	2,771
13-19	62.6	22.6	25.1	1,882
20+	61.7	16.6	20.2	825
Referred conditions				
0-1	67.7	24.9	24.1	4,686
2	66.1	24	23.7	2,482
3	65.8	21.6	23.4	1,679
	67.8	22.5	22	953

Table 11. (Continued)

	DOD Measure: Average answer exceeded neutral	GAO Measure: All answers positive		N
	Raw data	Raw data	Model estimates	
	Percentage	Percentage	Percentage	
DOD Percentage Rating				
0	66.5	20.8		236
10	67.3	24.6		1,287
20	66.6	23.1		978
30	67.1	23.7		680
40	67.2	22.2		531
50	65.4	21.5		786
60	66.7	23		609
70	68.2	21.2		556
80	68.9	30		280
90	63.1	21.3		122
100	75.5	35.5		282
MEB treatment facility				
Andrews	57.4	18.5	19.8	319
Lejeune	56.9	18	18.4	1,046
Pendleton	62.1	17	19.2	372
Belvoir	66.3	25	30.1	252
Benning	77.3	34	25.6	260
Bliss				0
Bragg	72.9	36.8	34.3	288
Campbell	90	50	47	10
Carson	64.3	19	23.7	736
Drum	67.3	30	27.9	397
Gordon	50	50		2
Hood	81.1	33.3	30.7	519
Lewis	59.5	21	20.2	252
Meade	55.5	15.6	14.7	218
Polk	81	33.3	28.1	400

	DOD Measure: Average answer exceeded neutral	GAO Measure: All answers positive		N
	Raw data	Raw data	Model estimates	
	Percentage	Percentage	Percentage	
Riley	59	20	17.4	105
Stewart	74.2	26.7	27	718
Other	68	25.6	20.3	961
Portsmouth	65	23	21.8	283
San Antonio	71.1	26.3	24.2	505
San Diego	65.2	20.5	21.3	1,127
Tripler	83.3	53	37.8	30
Walter Reed (Army)	65.2	21.7	26.4	511
Walter Reed (Navy/Marine	66.4	19.9	24.1	554
Time in IDES (GAO				
1st quartile	81.5	38.3	41.1	313
2nd quartile	78.2	35	33.8	1,658
3rd quartile	70.1	24.8	23.7	3,667
4th quartile	58.8	17.4	17.8	4,226
Sex				
Female	66.9	25.4	25.2	1,799
Male	67	23.5	23.3	8,063
Personnel Class				
Enlisted	67.1	23.9	23.9	9,126
Officer	64.5	21.7	21	691
Warrant	77	29.2	27.6	48
PEB Location				
Lewis	64.2	20.4		1,283
National Capital Region	66	26.1		1,698
San Antonio (Randolph)	61.8	23.6		838
San Antonio (Sam	76.5	30		2,417
Washington Navy Yard	63.1	19.9		3,629
MEB Exam Location				

Table 11. (Continued)

	DOD Measure: Average answer exceeded neutral	GAO Measure: All answers positive		N
	Raw data	Raw data	Model estimates	
	Percentage	Percentage	Percentage	
Military Treatment Facility	67.2	24.1	22.1	868
Contractor Facility	67	23.9	23.7	1,991
VA Medical Center	66.9	24.2	23.4	5,976
Not Available	66.9	21.2	27.2	1,030

Source: GAO analysis of DOD and VA data.

[a] Rollout phases correspond with the order in which IDES deployed at various facilities.

Specifically, the estimates are in-sample mean predicted probabilities of giving a satisfied response on the GAO satisfaction index from a logistic model of satisfaction. The covariates are given by indicators of whether the servicemember belonged to each group in column 4. The maximum likelihood estimators allowed the probability of satisfaction, given the covariates, to be dependent across observations within the 26 cross-classified groups of PEB location and MEB medical treatment facility. This adjusted for the possibility that servicemembers were similarly satisfied if they were processed in the same locations, given similar values on the observed covariates.[7]

Regardless of which measure is used (DOD's or GAO's), satisfaction varied only modestly across many important groups of servicemembers. Our model estimates that the GAO measure of satisfaction varied by no more than approximately five percentage points across branch, component, disenrollment outcome, sex, MEB exam provider, enlisted and officer personnel classes, and the number of claimed and referred conditions, although differences across MEB treatment facilities and PEB locations were larger.[8] This can be seen as a positive outcome, if this correlation implies that DOD and VA administer the program consistently across servicemembers and locations. However, the lack of variation also could suggest that the survey items do not measure opinions in enough detail to discriminate among servicemembers' experiences.

Also shown in table 11, satisfaction had a stronger association with case processing time (time spent in IDES) than some of the other factors we examined. Servicemembers whose case processing times were among the quickest 25 percent were about 2.3 times as likely to be satisfied (on the GAO scale) than those whose times were among the 25 percent of cases with the longest overall timeframes (i.e., 41 versus 18 percent). Nevertheless, only 41 percent of those servicemembers whose cases were processed most quickly were satisfied (holding constant the other factors). This suggests that servicemembers' opinions about IDES may be only loosely related to the amount of time they spent in IDES, as discussed in the next section below.

Although the average case processing time has generally increased since 2008, when we look at satisfaction by fiscal year, servicemember satisfaction shows evidence of improvement since fiscal year 2008. Specifically, our measure of satisfaction from the model increased by 15 percentage points since 2008, roughly doubling from 13 to 28. Because the model estimates control for various other factors, these results suggest that servicemember views of the IDES process have improved over time, rather than the possibility that IDES has simply processed different types of cases.

Satisfaction does not vary by a large amount across many MEB treatment facilities, but there are exceptions. Our model estimates that about 18 to 26 percent of servicemembers were satisfied at most facilities. However, there were pockets of greater satisfaction. Specifically, servicemembers had more positive experiences at Forts Belvoir, Bragg, Campbell, Drum, Hood, and Polk, with satisfaction estimated to have ranged from 28 to 45 percentage points. Fort Meade had the lowest satisfaction at 15 percent. These estimates hold constant time spent in IDES and other factors in column 4 and, thus, partially account for the types of cases each facility processes.

Satisfaction with Timeliness

DOD and VA measure IDES timeliness directly in VTA and as part of the overall servicemember satisfaction scale.

These overlapping measures let us compare servicemembers' opinions to their actual experiences in the program. To do this, we calculated processing times at each phase of IDES for servicemembers who expressed varying degrees of satisfaction with the timeliness of their case processing at that phase. In addition, we analyzed whether servicemembers who were satisfied with the overall IDES process were more or less likely to meet timeliness goals.

Table 12 provides these statistics. As shown in table 12, satisfaction generally stayed the same or decreased as processing times increased. The median days spent in the MEB and PEB phases were 35 and 38 percent lower, respectively, among those servicemembers who said that MEB and PEB timeliness was "very good" as compared to those who said it was "very poor."

Table 12. Perceived Timeliness of IDES by Actual Processing Times

	10th Pctile	*Days in IDES (by phase)* *Median*	*90th Pctile*	*Actual processing time (by Phase)* *% in 1st Quartile*	*% in 2nd Quartile*	*% in 3rd Quartile*	*% in 4th Quartile*	*% Met DOD Goal*	N
Overall satisfaction with IDES (GAO Measure)									
Not satisfied	198	348	544	2.57	14.33	36.68	46.42	33.8	7,516
Satisfied	159	297	479	5.11	24.74	38.76	31.39	50.2	2,349
Perceived MEB timeliness									
Very poor	88	175	323	7.9	22.5	30.9	38.7	16.8	1,685
Poor	78	156	290	11.6	25.7	35.1	27.6	23.4	1,594
Mix of poor/good	72	142	273	15.1	28.6	34.7	21.6	27.9	2,397
Good	66	128	254	19.8	31.9	29.8	18.6	35.6	2,811
Very good	62	114	223	24.9	38.2	24.3	12.6	45.3	1,200
Perceived PEB timeliness satisfaction									
Very poor	28	88	203	22.8	18.1	23.7	35.4	67.8	759
Poor	28	89	186	20.8	18.9	24.7	35.7	69.7	680
Mix of poor/good	23	70	155	28.3	23.4	24	24.3	79.5	1,262
Good	23	65	138	30.7	25.5	24.4	19.4	84.3	1,470
Very good	17	55	128	40.2	26.2	18	15.6	88.1	740
Perceived Transition timeliness									
Very poor	33	87	461	7.9	22.5	30.9	38.7	16.1	500
Poor	43	90	459	11.6	25.7	35.1	27.6	12.6	468
Mix of poor/good	40	90	481	15.1	28.6	34.7	21.6	13.3	967
Good	37	91	496	19.8	31.9	29.8	18.6	12.8	1,065
Very good	39	91	657	24.9	38.2	24.3	12.6	12.8	541

Source: GAO analysis of DOD and VA data.

The former group was 170 percent more likely to have met the MEB timeliness goal and 30 percent more likely to have met the PEB timeliness goal. Similarly, the case for a median servicemember—whom we classified as "satisfied" with the overall IDES process—was completed 15 percent more quickly and was 49 percent more likely to have met the timeliness goal than the median servicemember who was "dissatisfied." The model estimates in table 11 confirm that the GAO measure of satisfaction and timeliness (time spent in IDES) are negatively related even when holding constant several other variables.

Perceived and actual timeliness had little association at the Transition phase. Across all levels of satisfaction with timeliness, the median processing time varied by no more than 4 days, and the proportion meeting the timeliness goal varied by no more than 4 percentage points. The use of personal leave is one plausible explanation for the unresponsiveness of servicemember satisfaction to actual processing times in the Transition phase. A servicemember might not have been dissatisfied with delays if taking leave was the reason, rather than the IDES process itself. Despite the associations between actual and perceived timeliness at the MEB and PEB phases, there were many servicemembers who were satisfied or dissatisfied with timeliness that spent similar amounts of time in the program. For example, 68 percent of those who said that PEB timeliness was "very poor" completed the phase on time, and 55 percent of those who said that MEB timeliness was "very good" did not complete on time.

Among servicemembers who said that MEB timeliness was "very good," the middle 80 percent of processing times ranged from 62 days to 223 days. The same range for servicemembers who said MEB timeliness was "very poor" was 88 to 323 days. As table 12 shows, a similar pattern holds for the PEB phase.

Although servicemembers tend to be more satisfied in MEB and PEB when their cases take less time, many of them are highly dissatisfied even when their cases take an unusually short amount of time (and vice versa). In the Transition phase, however, 40 percent of servicemembers who said that timeliness was "very good" were processed in 91 to 657 days—a more lengthy range than at the other phases.

The large range and relationship with satisfaction may reflect the use of servicemember leave. The fact that many servicemembers are similarly satisfied with timeliness, even though they can have widely different processing times, has broader implications for measuring the performance of IDES. DOD's timeliness goals may not be meaningful to servicemembers or necessarily reflect high-quality service. Alternatively, servicemembers may not use reasonable standards to assess the time required to process their cases, or they may not accurately perceive the time they have spent in the program. In these scenarios, the value of servicemember satisfaction as a performance measure becomes less certain.

The relationship between perceived and actual timeliness may simply reflect a large amount of unobserved heterogeneity across servicemembers. For example, a servicemember whose case has been in IDES for an extremely long time might still be highly satisfied with timeliness if the case was complex or personal leave was taken during the process. Neither the survey nor the VTA data measure these or other such characteristics that might affect the program's key performance measures.

Factors Affecting Survey Results and Implications for Program Evaluation

The lack of variation in satisfaction across servicemember groups and according case timeliness might be seen as a positive outcome, and may suggest that DOD and VA administer the program consistently across servicemembers and locations. However, the lack of variation also could suggest shortcomings in the design and administration of the survey, or in data limitations that, alone or together, may reduce the usefulness of survey data for program evaluation. For example:

- *Survey questions*: The survey questions may not be sufficiently detailed to measure important differences among servicemembers' experiences. For example, the survey includes 12 questions (4 per survey) that measure broad opinions about IDES, and DOD subsequently averages these responses together. This approach may limit the survey's capacity to describe IDES experiences in sufficient detail.
- *Precision of DOD indices*: DOD reports measures of overall satisfaction with IDES for each phase, using the questions in table 9. However, these measures include one question that asks respondents to "evaluate their overall experience since entering the IDES process," which could be influenced by experiences in prior phases. Consequently, the satisfaction measures reported for each phase could

represent a combination of servicemembers' experiences in that phase and prior phases.

- Completing two surveys at once: DOD officials told us that a servicemember may be surveyed for the PEB and Transition phases in one session. In these instances a large amount of time may have passed since the servicemember completed the PEB phase and it may be more difficult for the servicemember to isolate his or her satisfaction with a particular phase.
- Survey design: The satisfaction survey is primarily designed to measure performance, not explain it. The survey includes many highly correlated questions measuring satisfaction with the overall process or broad components of it, such as DOD board liaisons, VA case managers, or timeliness. While multiple questions can improve the statistical reliability and validity of DOD's performance measures, they require costly survey administration time that could be used for other purposes, such as to measure a larger number of variables that could explain servicemember satisfaction or case processing times.
- VTA data limitations: The VTA administrative data that we matched to survey data primarily measure processing times and basic servicemember demographics, such as service branch, component, and treatment facility. The data support detailed reporting of performance measures, but they do not measure similarly detailed information on the nature of each case that might allow DOD and VA to understand the reasons for lengthy case processing times or to identify cases that might become delayed and ensure that they remain on schedule. For example, the database does not measure the type or severity of referred medical conditions in detail, the nature of delays experienced early in the process, or the use of servicemember leave. In addition, little information is available on staffing at or caseloads for MEB and PEB locations, DOD board liaisons, or VA case managers, which might help to explain or predict performance.
- Low response and coverage rates: The response and coverage rates of the satisfaction survey further limit the degree to which DOD can generalize the data obtained to the population of servicemembers who participate in IDES. In particular, the survey does not assess the views of servicemembers who disenroll from the process before finishing a stage or those who do not complete prior waves of the survey. Including servicemembers who do not complete all waves would complicate longitudinal analysis, however.

APPENDIX III: MONTHLY DOD TIMELINESS DATA FOR ACTIVE DUTY CASES IN FISCAL YEAR 2012

Table 13 presents data reported by DOD on average processing time for active duty cases completed during part of fiscal year 2012—Oct. 2011 to June 2012. DOD's data are provided as a supplement the analyses GAO conducted for fiscal years 2008 through 2011.1 We did not evaluate the reliability of these data and cannot predict the extent to which any trends will continue for the rest of the fiscal year.

Table 13. DOD Reported Monthly Average Processing Times for Active Component Servicemembers in Fiscal Year 2012 (in days)

				Month that IDES process, phase or stage was completed						
Time spent in:	Goal (days)	Oct. 2011	Nov. 2011	Dec. 2011	Jan. 2012	Feb. 2012	Mar. 2012	Apr. 2012	May 2012	June 2012
IDES overall (only cases resulting in receipt of benefits)	295	395	391	404	395	392	394	400	409	395
MEB phase	100	136	130	128	132	130	124	114	116	122
Medical Exam Stage	45	40	39	41	44	37	37	39	39	39
MEB Stage	35	76	71	73	76	77	72	64	66	69
PEB phase	120	95	100	104	112	116	111	114	120	122
Informal PEB stage	15	23	28	34	34	28	23	22	19	24
VA Preliminary Rating stage	15	26	27	31	34	37	51	58	45	35
Transition phase	45	71	70	69	75	77	76	74	77	74
VA Benefits phase	30	38	36	47	56	49	50	57	66	62

Source: DOD IDES Monthly Reports for April, May June , and July 2012.

Note: This table does not reflect data on all phases or stages of the IDES process. Instead, it presents data on those phases and stages that GAO also presented data on in the body of the report.

End Notes

[1] GAO, Military and Veterans Disability System: Pilot Has Achieved Some Goals, but Further Planning and Monitoring Needed, GAO-11-69 (Washington, D.C.: Dec. 6, 2010).

[2] We visited the facilities at Joint Base Andrews and Fort Meade, Maryland; Naval Hospital Bremerton and Joint Base Lewis-McChord (Madigan Army Medical Center), Washington; and Forts Hood and Sam Houston, Texas.

[3] A physician is required to identify a condition that may cause the member to fall below retention standards after the member has received the maximum benefit of medical care.

[4] In this report, "DOD board liaisons" refers to DOD Physical Evaluation Board Liaison Officers, while "VA case managers" refers to VA Military Service Coordinators.

[5] This evaluation is based on the results of the medical exams, the member's medical records, and input from the member's commanding officer.

[6] VA determines the degree to which veterans are disabled in 10 percent increments on a scale of 0 to 100 percent. If VA finds that a veteran has one or more service-connected disabilities with a combined rating of at least 10 percent, the agency will pay monthly compensation.

[7] The reviewing authorities of PEBs in the respective services are the Air Force Personnel Council, the Army Physical Disability Agency, and the Navy Council of Review Boards.

[8] The three original pilot sites were Walter Reed Army Medical Center, Washington, D.C.; National Naval Medical Center, Bethesda, Maryland; and Malcolm Grow Air Force Medical Center, Andrews Air Force Base.

[9] When processing times are broken down by the year of completion, as in Figure 4, the average processing times in the first few years are lower since cases with longer processing times after the program's inception in fiscal year 2008 would not show up in the data until fiscal year 2009 or later.

[10] Our data were for cases in the MEB phase as of December 31, 2011. For cases that had not yet been in the MEB for 100 days (the MEB goal), we cannot predict whether they will be timely cases or not. For instance some of these cases entered the MEB phase just days before the cutoff date GAO chose.

[11] As previously noted, the narrative summary documents the medical conditions and the impact of these conditions on the servicemembers' ability to perform their military duties.

[12] VA's goal is 1 case manager for every 30 new cases.

[13] DOD did not provide monthly data on the percentage of reservist cases meeting these stage goals. See app. III for more information on monthly processing times.

[14] According to VA officials, reservists who are not on active duty do not have a transition phase.

[15] DOD and VA did not set a goal for reserve component servicemembers. As noted above, for purposes of this report, we opted to not include reserve component time spent in the VA benefit phase in our calculations phase because this goal applies to some but not all reservists, depending on their active duty status. Any time spent within the VA benefit phase is reflected within the overall processing time calculations for such reserve component servicemembers.

[16] DOD officials also told us that a servicemember may be surveyed simultaneously for a prior phase along with the phase just completed (e.g. the MEB and PEB phases). However, in some cases a significant amount of time may have passed since the servicemember completed the prior phase and, thus, it may be more difficult for the servicemember to isolate his or her satisfaction with a particular phase.

[17] DOD could interview a probability sample of servicemembers to accurately assess satisfaction with IDES in the population as a whole. A sample could decrease the cost of obtaining this information, because DOD would need to contact fewer servicemembers and the cost of surveys generally increases with the number of people interviewed. If properly designed and executed, a probability sample would provide estimates that would be equally valid as interviewing all servicemembers.

[18] Using DOD's satisfaction measure, we found less than expected variation in satisfaction over time and across key case characteristics, such as component, military branch, final rating and final disposition. To better understand factors that may drive servicemember satisfaction, we included neutral responses in the category of "not satisfied" rather than counting such responses as "satisfied" in the manner that DOD did thus arriving at a measure that more strongly reflects satisfaction and might be a more sensitive indicator of factors affecting satisfaction for performance management purposes.

[19] Military Disability System: Increased Supports for Servicemembers and Better Pilot Planning Could Improve the Disability Evaluation Process, GAO-08-1137 (Washington, D.C.: Sept. 24, 2008).

[20] In January 2012, senior agency officials decided to merge the DOD-VA Senior Oversight Committee into the DOD-VA Joint Executive Council, co-chaired by the Under Secretary of Defense (Personnel and Readiness) and the Deputy Secretary of Veterans Affairs. DOD and VA plan to establish a joint IDES working group under the Joint Executive Council. Meanwhile, the IDES has been incorporated into the agencies' Joint Strategic Plan, and agency stakeholders meet weekly to discuss IDES issues.

[21] The Army has physicians dedicated to MEB cases. In contrast, Navy and Air Force MEB determinations are prepared by physicians who perform other responsibilities, such as clinical treatment and supervision.

[22] Originally, reserve component members determined to require IDES referral were referred to the MEB at Fort Gordon, Georgia. According to Army officials, these members are referred to one of 10 Army MEBs.

[23] A DOD official told us that based on recent negative feedback, including from site visits, DOD is considering cancelling this pilot project.

[24] As of March 2012, the Seattle rating site is responsible for cases from all 3 Army PEBs.

[25] Under this proposed process, VA would not begin work on a case until a servicemember was found to be unfit for military service by an informal PEB. The pilot was postponed in response to concerns raised by the military services and VA about specific changes to the existing process. For example, VA officials expressed concerns that the preliminary VA rating could occur long after the servicemember was found to be unfit for duty, which could cause the servicemember to seek a formal PEB hearing.

[26] In January and February 2012, teams visited Little Rock Air Force Base, Arkansas; Naval Medical Center San Diego, California; Fort Carson, Colorado; Wright-Patterson Air Force Base, Ohio; and Naval Medical Center Portsmouth, Virginia. In March 2012, a team visited Joint Base Andrews, Maryland, and Fort Eustis and Naval Health Clinic Quantico, Virginia, to examine the piloting of a new DOD-wide IDES information system.

[27] The original facilities were Walter Reed Army Medical Center, National Naval Medical Center, Brooke Army Medical Center (Fort Sam Houston), and Naval Medical Center San Diego.

End Notes for Appendix I

[1] DOD's Office of Warrior Care Policy changed its name from the Office of Wounded Warrior Care and Transition Policy (WWCTP) in 2012.

[2] The number of active and Reserve components cases do not add up to the number of total cases because seven cases did not have a component code in the data.

[3] Demographic data included such information as gender, personnel class, service branch, component, and the number of conditions claimed and referred.

[4] GAO, Military and Veterans Disability System: Pilot Has Achieved Some Goals, but Further Planning and Monitoring Needed, GAO-11-69 (Washington, D.C.: Dec. 6, 2010).

[5] Our analysis found an additional 11 percent of cases with dates missing for stages in the IDES program—dates that were not critical to our analyses. We believe that many if not most of these cases of missing data might be explainable. Servicemembers do not always pass through every step of the process and we believe this may explain some portion of missing dates. However, without looking at case files for all of these cases or the VTA data in more detail we cannot determine what portion of those 11 percent have a reasonable explanation for being missing.

[6] We did not review the data on a monthly basis because this is done in DOD's monthly reports and we wanted to provide a longer term perspective of the evolution of the IDES program.

[7] While we have data through December for fiscal year 2012, we did not include these data in our analysis because we sought to compare completed fiscal years.

[8] Including Directive-Type Memorandum 11-015, which establishes policies, assigns responsibilities, and prescribes procedures for the IDES.

End Notes for Appendix II

[1] We consider processing times overall, for the four phases of IDES (MEB, PEB, Transition, and VA Benefits), Active Duty, Reserve, or National Guard status, and for servicemembers receiving benefits versus all servicemembers regardless of the outcome of their cases.

[2] Response rates refer to the percentages of servicemen who responded to the surveys among those who DOD deemed eligible. For the MEB survey, eligibles included all servicemen who completed the MEB phase, but for the PEB and Transition surveys eligibles included only those who completed those phases and also completed the prior surveys. Coverage rates refer the percentages of servicemen that responded to each survey among those who completed each phase, regardless of whether they completed prior surveys.

[3] GAO's latest data export from the VTA database included data through January 1, 2012.

[4] The servicemembers included in these figures have not necessarily completed the entire IDES process, but did complete a given phase to be included in the figure for that phase.

[5] Though there are different ways to calculate response and coverage rates, which can result in different estimates of these quantities, we chose our response rate and coverage estimates in order to better understand what fraction of the intended group was actually surveyed.

[6] Both measures of satisfaction combine responses from servicemembers who have finished various phases of IDES. For example, a servicemember who completed only the MEB would provide at most 4 responses from that wave's survey, while a servicemember who completed all phases would provide at most 12 responses from all three surveys. Each measure calculates overall satisfaction using all responses available, even though the number of responses varies among servicemembers (e.g., 4 vs. 12).

[7] Because the "cluster-robust" variance estimator is only consistent as the number of clusters becomes large, the relatively small number of MEB-PEB locations in our data raises the possibility of finite-sample bias. The practical effect of this problem should be minimal, however, since the model controls for MEB and PEB location and, thus, residual intraclass correlation should be small.

[8] In addition, servicemembers who were found unfit and returned to duty—a rare outcome—were approximately 4 to 10 percentage points less likely to be satisfied than servicemembers who had any of the other outcomes.

End Note for Appendix III

[1] DOD calculates timeliness separately for active, reserve, and guard components. Because our report includes analysis for active and reserve/guard combined, we are only including active servicemembers in this appendix for easy comparison. Active duty cases reflect the bulk of cases in fiscal year 2012, as with other fiscal years.

INDEX

A

B

C

S

T

U

V

W

Y